HEART FAILURE: CURRENT CLINICAL UNDERSTANDING

George C Sutton & Kanu Chatterjee

Published by Remedica

Commonwealth House, 1 New Oxford Street, London, WC1A 1NU, UK

Civic Opera Building, 20 North Wacker Drive, Suite 1642, Chicago, IL 60606, USA

info@remedicabooks.com

www.remedicabooks.com

Tel: +44 (0)20 7759 2999

Fax: +44 (0)20 7759 2951

Publisher: Andrew Ward

In-house editors: Catherine Booth and Carolyn Dunn

Design and Artwork: AS&K Skylight Creative Services

© 2008 Remedica

Remedica is a member of the AS&K Media Partnership.

ISBN: 978 1 901346 97 8

British Library Cataloguing-in-Publication Data.

A catalogue record for this book is available from the British Library.

Printed in the UK

HEART FAILURE: CURRENT CLINICAL UNDERSTANDING

George C Sutton, MD, FRCP (Lond), FACC

Senior Lecturer in Cardiology
National Heart and Lung Institute
Imperial College London

Kanu Chatterjee, MD, FRCP (Lond), FRCP (Edin), FCCP, FACC, MACP

Ernest Gallo Distinguished Professor of Medicine
Division of Cardiology
University of California, San Francisco Medical Center

Acknowledgments

The authors gratefully acknowledge Eli Botvinick, William Ong, Dana McGlothlin, and Curtis Looney of University of California, San Francisco, and Mary Sheppard of the Royal Brompton Hospital for providing many of the illustrations.

Acknowledgment is also extended to all the people who contributed to *Clinical Cardiology: An Illustrated Text* written also by George C Sutton and Kanu Chatterjee. Some of the material included in this book also appeared in that title.

Preface

Heart failure is usually the end stage of any heart disease. Because heart disease is common, the prevalence and incidence of heart failure are high, and heart failure is one of the most frequent reasons for admission to hospital. As the treatment of heart disease improves, patients are surviving for longer, and those who develop heart failure are usually elderly.

This illustrated text aims to provide an up-to-date account of the diagnosis, epidemiology, management, and prognosis of heart failure. It is not intended to be a chapter from a textbook of medicine or cardiology, but rather a way of understanding heart failure for clinicians who see and manage patients with this clinical syndrome. It is written for undergraduate and postgraduate students of medicine, general and care-of-the-elderly physicians, primary care physicians, and trainees in cardiology.

Although the diagnostic aspects of heart failure have changed relatively little in recent years, there has been an increase in knowledge of its epidemiology and prognosis. Management has changed most of all, and the section on this aspect of heart failure is designed to reflect the current situation using an evidence-based approach.

Many cardiologists have influenced our own thinking on heart failure. We owe all of them our thanks. We would like especially to thank our wives, Jane and Docey, for their support and stimulus during the writing of this text.

George C Sutton

Kanu Chatterjee

Foreword

Today textbooks are read less than they were in the past. This is because so many patients, health workers, and doctors obtain much information from the Internet. The difficulty is that such a morass of information is available that it is often impossible for the untrained or non-specialist to determine what to believe and just what significance to attach to any statement. Additionally, the surfeit of data can create a nightmare of uncertainty and anxiety for the patient. The solution is good doctoring: the physician should have the trust of the patient, and should explain the medical condition and the necessary investigations in language that can be readily understood. However, this is made challenging for doctors because they are overwhelmed with guidelines, particularly in the field of heart failure. While adherence to guidelines, in general, does improve patients' outcomes, too much of an obsession with guidelines and protocols can have the disadvantage of reducing professionalism and, rather than providing personalized medicine, imposing dictums.

This book goes someway to restoring professionalism in the treatment of heart failure. It is written by two distinguished experts with years of clinical experience who were trained in an era when more attention was paid to clinical observation and clinical skills than it is today. The directness of the text reflects the broad knowledge and confidence of these two cardiologists, and the book is easy to read, a quality becoming ever rarer. The text is also accompanied by illustrations that are both relevant and useful. The book will be invaluable to students, primary care physicians, health workers, and cardiovascular physicians.

Philip A Poole-Wilson, MB, MD, FRCP, FMedSci
Professor of Cardiology
British Heart Foundation Simon Marks Chair of Cardiology
National Heart & Lung Institute
Imperial College London

Foreword

The importance of heart failure as a public health problem throughout the world has become evident to just about everyone who is involved in health care. Heart failure is pandemic in industrialized nations and its prevalence is increasing rapidly in developing countries. The expectation is that the worldwide burden of impaired quality of life, loss of earning power, increased health care costs (in particular, those related to hospitalization), and premature mortality due to heart failure will increase substantially over the next several decades.

Fortunately, over recent years we have made considerable progress in both our understanding of the pathophysiology of heart failure and the way we treat patients with this condition. With the increase in availability of effective therapies, selection of the most appropriate treatment strategy for an individual patient has become much more complicated. While heart failure therapy may not be as individualized as cancer therapy, there is no question of there being a rote formula for deciding how to manage each patient optimally, and there is no single therapeutic approach that is applicable to all heart failure patients.

This beautifully illustrated text provides an authoritative presentation of the current knowledge base on heart failure from a clinically relevant perspective. Moreover, the material is presented in a manner that is understandable to non-specialists in the area. Readers will be treated to an overview of the best management strategies currently available, together with practical information and examples that will help to put these approaches into the context of the specific patient. With this knowledge, the advances in management can be more fully translated into improved outcomes in our patients, which ultimately is our primary goal.

Barry Greenberg, MD
Professor of Medicine
Director, Advanced Heart Failure Treatment Program
University of California, San Diego

Contents

Diagnosis   1

Epidemiology   30

Management   34

Prognosis   48

References   51

Abbreviations   54

Index   55

Diagnosis

Although a number of definitions of heart failure have been proposed, there is no uniform definition. "A condition in which the heart fails to discharge its contents adequately" was proposed by Sir Thomas Lewis in 1933 [1]. Other definitions have included: "Heart failure is a complex clinical syndrome that can result from any structural or functional cardiac disorder that impairs the ability of the ventricle to fill with or eject blood" [2]; "A pathophysiological state in which an abnormality of cardiac function is responsible for the failure of the heart to pump blood at a rate commensurate with the requirements of the metabolizing tissues" [3]; and "A clinical syndrome caused by an abnormality of the heart and recognized by a characteristic pattern of hemodynamic, renal, neural, and hormonal responses" [4].

These definitions provide insight into the pathophysiologic mechanisms that are a feature of heart failure, but they are difficult to use in clinical practice. In order for the clinician to determine whether the individual patient has heart failure, a definition that can be applied clinically is required. Such a definition has been proposed by the Task Force for Heart Failure of the European Society of Cardiology: "Symptoms of heart failure (at rest or on exercise) and objective evidence of cardiac dysfunction at rest" [5]. Whereas all the definitions emphasize that in order to have heart failure the patient must have evidence of a cardiac abnormality, the European Society's definition emphasizes that the patient's symptoms must be consistent with the clinical diagnosis of heart failure.

Symptoms and signs

The most frequent symptom of heart failure is breathlessness (dyspnea). Breathlessness is common to all types of heart failure. It can manifest as paroxysmal nocturnal dyspnea (breathlessness that wakes the patient at night), orthopnea (breathlessness when lying flat), or dyspnea on exertion. The other key symptom, particularly in patients with chronic heart failure, is fatigue.

Signs that are consistent with the diagnosis of heart failure include features that result from activation of the neurohormonal systems: these include fluid retention (either pulmonary or peripheral edema) and elevation of the jugular venous pressure (**Figure 1**). Sinus tachycardia and peripheral vasoconstriction result from activation of the sympathetic nervous system. However, the presence of such abnormal symptoms and physical signs alone does not permit the diagnosis of heart failure in the individual patient: in addition, there must be evidence of a cardiac abnormality.

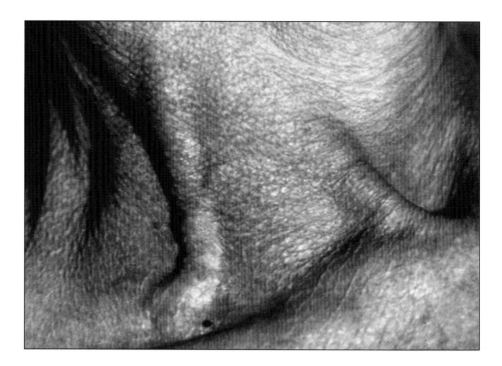

Figure 1. Distended external jugular vein in a patient with chronic heart failure.

Cardiac abnormalities

Evidence of a cardiac abnormality may be obtained from examination of the cardiovascular system. Because any cardiac abnormality can lead to the clinical syndrome of heart failure, abnormal physical signs can vary from evidence of left ventricular (LV) myocardial dysfunction (double apical impulse on palpation of the precordium, third and fourth heart sounds [**Figure 2**], summation gallops on auscultation, and a pansystolic murmur due to secondary atrioventricular valve regurgitation) to the auscultatory features of primary valve disease (eg, mitral stenosis) or congenital heart disease.

However, the presence of such abnormal cardiac signs in isolation does not indicate that the patient has heart failure unless there are additional symptoms (notably dyspnea) and physical signs (notably edema), as outlined above. Abnormal cardiac signs without symptoms simply indicate that the patient has a cardiac abnormality, but not clinically overt heart failure.

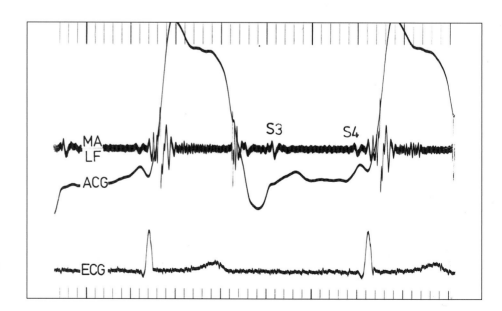

Figure 2. Simultaneous phonocardiogram (recorded in the mitral area at low-frequency [MA-LF]), apex cardiogram (ACG), and electrocardiogram (ECG) to show the third (S3) and fourth (S4) heart sounds. S3 coincides with the peak of the rapid filling wave in the ACG, while S4 coincides with the peak of the 'a' wave (due to atrial contraction) in the ACG.

A cardiac abnormality may be detected not only by the presence of abnormal findings on examination, but also by a variety of invasive and noninvasive investigations of the heart. These include the electrocardiogram (ECG), echocardiography and Doppler imaging, nuclear imaging, magnetic resonance imaging (MRI), computed tomography (CT) imaging, cardiac catheterization, angiography, and myocardial biopsy. These are discussed further in the **Investigations** section.

PATHOPHYSIOLOGY

Any cardiac abnormality can give rise to heart failure. Pathologic conditions of the heart include those involving myocardial, pericardial, valvular, or congenital disease (**Figures 3–7**). LV myocardial disease is the most common pathologic abnormality to give rise to heart failure. Myocardial dysfunction is most frequently the result of coronary artery disease (CAD), and forms the main substrate for the development of heart failure. Such myocardial dysfunction may be associated with either a reduced or preserved LV ejection fraction (EF)

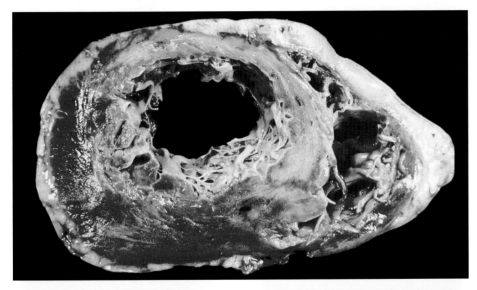

Figure 3. Transverse slice of the ventricles. A recent full-thickness myocardial infarction is present in the anterior wall of the left ventricle extending into the interventricular septum.

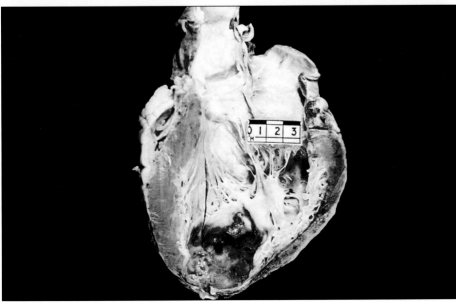

Figure 4. Localized left ventricular aneurysm due to previous myocardial infarction. The aneurysm contains a fine deposit of thrombus and a large central cavity opening into the ventricle.

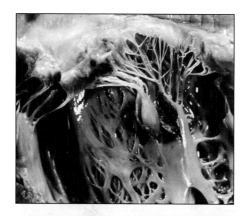

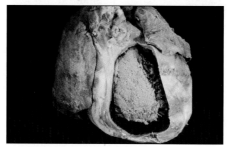

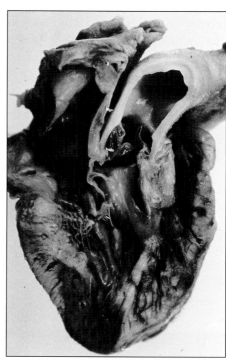

Figure 5 (top). Partial avulsion of a papillary muscle as a result of acute myocardial infarction. One head of the postero-medial papillary muscle is torn from the ventricular wall.

Figure 6 (bottom). Chronic constrictive pericarditis. A window has been cut through the thickened parietal pericardium which forms a rough constrictive membrane. There is a shaggy exudate on the visceral pericardium.

Figure 7 (right). Right ventricular view in tetralogy of Fallot. The aorta overrides the ventricular septal defect, and the infundibular septum is deviated anteriorly to produce infundibular pulmonary stenosis.

(see the next sections). The pathologic changes that occur in the myocardium are termed "LV remodeling". Although remodeling occurs irrespective of whether the EF remains preserved or reduced, the changes are different in the two situations.

Remodeling with reduced ejection fraction

In cases of heart failure due to myocardial dysfunction in which the EF is reduced (**Table 1**), the left ventricle is dilated and becomes spherical in shape. This change in shape is the main factor contributing to the development of secondary mitral regurgitation, which further increases ventricular volumes. LV wall thickness is normal or reduced (**Figures 8** and **9**). Although there is a significant increase in LV mass, the cavity:mass ratio is markedly increased due to a disproportionate increase in LV cavity size. As a result, there is a substantial increase in LV wall stress, which contributes to the reduced EF. Reduced EF also results from decreased contractile function.

Mechanical dyssynchrony, with or without electrical dyssynchrony, is present in approximately 30% of patients and contributes further to the impairment in systolic function. Mechanical dyssynchrony is characterized by asynchronous contraction and relaxation of different myocardial segments.

Table 1. Pathophysiology of heart failure with reduced ejection fraction.

Altered ventricular shape and geometry
Normal or reduced left ventricular wall thickness
Disproportionate increase in ventricular cavity size
Increased ventricular mass
Increased cavity:mass ratio
Increased wall stress
Reduced contractile function
Reduced ejection fraction
Frequent mechanical dyssynchrony, with or without electrical dyssynchrony

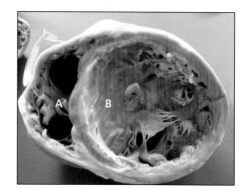

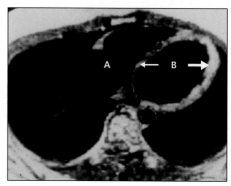

Figure 8 (left). Transverse section of right (A) and left ventricle (B) in dilated cardiomyopathy. The left ventricle is scarred with an increase in cavity size. The wall thickness of the left ventricle is reduced.

Courtesy of M. Sheppard, Royal Brompton Hospital, London.

Figure 9 (right). Magnetic resonance image (long axis view) of left (B) and right (A) ventricles in ischemic dilated cardiomyopathy. The left ventricle is dilated and spherical in shape. The thickness of the anterior wall of the left ventricle (thick arrow) is normal and the septal thickness (thin arrow) is decreased.

Eccentric hypertrophy is the dominant feature in heart failure with reduced EF, although in dilated cardiomyopathy, which is the result of CAD, concentric hypertrophy may also occur. Eccentric hypertrophy is characterized by lengthening of the myocytes with very little change in their width, resulting in an increase in length:width ratio (**Figure 10**) [6]. Comparllowing the ventricle to dilate. LV biopsy has shown that the myocyte diameter and myofibrillar density are lower in systolic heart failure than in diastolic heart failure [7].

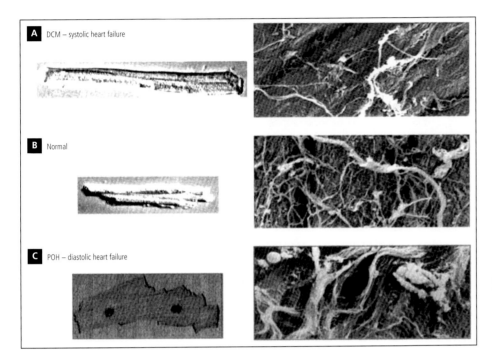

A — DCM – systolic heart failure

B — Normal

C — POH – diastolic heart failure

Figure 10. Studies in animal models of changes in length and width of the myocytes in a normal heart (B), in heart failure with reduced ejection fraction (systolic heart failure) due to dilated cardiomyopathy (DCM) (A), and in heart failure with preserved ejection fraction (diastolic heart failure) resulting from hypertrophy due to pressure overload (POH) (C).

Reproduced with permission from Lippincott Williams and Wilkins (Aurigemma GP, Zile MR, Gasch WH. Contractile behavior of the left ventricle in diastolic heart falure. *Circulation* 2006;113:296–304).

The biochemical, cellular, and molecular mechanisms of remodeling have also been studied. Calcium regulation, which controls contraction and relaxation of the myocytes, is abnormal. The extracellular matrix architecture is also abnormal. In cases of heart failure due to myocardial disease with reduced EF, the molecular mechanisms are characterized by an increased ratio of matrix metalloproteinase (MMP) to tissue inhibitor of metalloproteinase (TIMP). The collagen cross-links are decreased and the concentration of titin isoforms, which contribute to maintaining the compliance and stiffness of the ventricle, is also altered [8].

Specific remodeling features can be seen in patients in whom heart failure with reduced EF is due to CAD. Soon after a significant acute myocardial infarction (MI), the infarcted segments expand due to stretching and thinning. In the infarcted segments, there is myocyte necrosis and disruption of the extracellular architecture. In the myocardial segments remote from the infarcted areas, myocyte loss continues due to necrosis and apoptosis. There is also concurrent disruption of the extracellular collagen matrix, allowing these segments to stretch and the left ventricle to dilate (**Figure 11**).

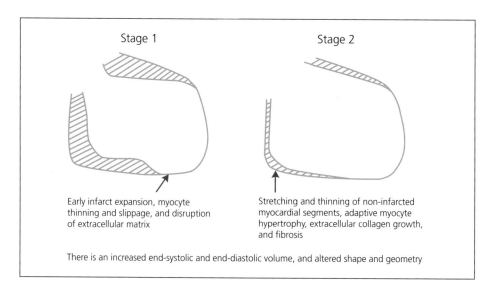

Stage 1

Stage 2

Early infarct expansion, myocyte thinning and slippage, and disruption of extracellular matrix

Stretching and thinning of non-infarcted myocardial segments, adaptive myocyte hypertrophy, extracellular collagen growth, and fibrosis

There is an increased end-systolic and end-diastolic volume, and altered shape and geometry

Figure 11. Schematic illustration of left ventricular remodeling soon after acute myocardial infarction (Stage 1) and late after myocardial infarction (Stage 2).

Remodeling with preserved ejection fraction

In cases of heart failure due to myocardial disease with preserved EF, ventricular remodeling has distinctive features that contrast with those seen in patients with reduced EF (**Table 2**). The LV chamber size is usually normal, occasionally even reduced in size, and is rarely dilated unless there have been episodes of MI or myocardial ischemia. There is concentric hypertrophy, and an increase in LV wall thickness (**Figure 12**) [6]. The cavity:mass ratio is uniformly decreased.

Table 2. Pathophysiology of heart failure with preserved ejection fraction.

| Normal or slight reduction in ventricular cavity size |
| Concentric ventricular hypertrophy |
| Increased wall thickness |
| Decreased cavity:mass ratio |
| Decreased wall stress |
| Normal ejection fraction |
| Little or no change in ventricular shape |
| Mechanical dyssynchrony may be present even in absence of wide QRS |

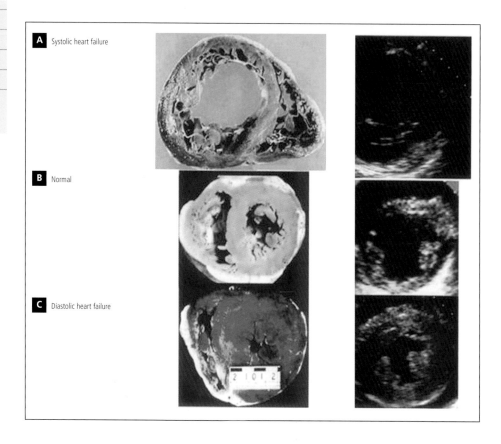

Figure 12. The left hand panel shows a transverse section of the right and left ventricle in a normal heart (B), and in severe heart failure with reduced (systolic heart failure, A) and preserved (diastolic heart failure, C) ejection fraction. In the right hand panel, two-dimensional echocardiographic cross-sectional views of the right and left ventricle are shown. The same comparative appearances can be seen as in the autopsy specimens.

Reproduced with permission from Lippincott Williams and Wilkins (Aurigemma GP, Zile MR, Gasch WH. Contractile behavior of the left ventricle in diastolic heart failure. *Circulation* 2006;113:296–304).

The increased LV wall thickness, together with decreased wall stress, maintains a normal EF. There is seldom alteration of the ventricular shape. Mechanical dyssynchrony may be present in approximately 30% of patients, even in the absence of a wide QRS complex in the ECG.

The width of the myocytes is markedly increased without any change in length, resulting in a decrease in the length:width ratio. There is increased extracellular collagen volume and fibrosis, but the collagen fibrillar bundles are thicker (**Figure 10**) and their maintained continuity prevents significant dilatation of the left ventricle.

The tissue expressions of the MMPs are decreased and that of the TIMPs increased, resulting in increased collagen synthesis and fibrosis, which together contribute to increased myocardial stiffness. In advanced heart failure with preserved EF, myocyte loss is increased by both necrosis and apoptosis. A comparison of the principal differences in the pathophysiology of remodeling with reduced and preserved EF is shown in **Table 3**.

Table 3. Differences in remodeling in heart failure with reduced ejection fraction (REF) or preserved ejection fraction (PEF). EDV: end-diastolic volume; ESV: end-systolic volume.

	REF	PEF
Hypertrophy	Eccentric	Concentric
EDV	Increased	Normal
ESV	Increased	Normal
Ejection fraction	Decreased	Normal
Dyssynchrony	May be present	May be present
Fibrosis	Increased	Increased
Apoptosis	Present	Present
Necrosis	Present	Present

The major functional abnormality in patients with overt heart failure due to myocardial disease with preserved EF is increased LV passive stiffness and decreased LV compliance, which is associated with an upward shift of the diastolic pressure–volume curve. Thus, there is a disproportionate increase in LV diastolic pressure for any increment in diastolic volume (**Figure 13**) [9]. With a marked upward and leftward shift of the diastolic pressure–volume curve, the stroke volume may also decrease without any change in contractile function (**Figure 14**) [10].

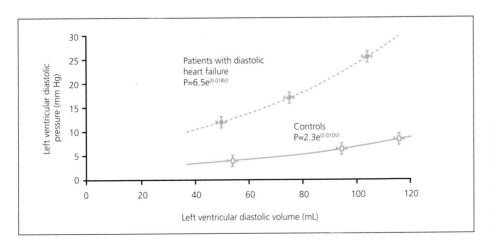

Patients with diastolic heart failure
$P=6.5e^{(0.018V)}$

Controls
$P=2.3e^{(0.010V)}$

Figure 13. Diastolic pressure–volume relation in patients with heart failure with preserved ejection fraction and in controls. The figure shows measured values for the minimal left ventricular pressure (P = stiffness constant). The data indicate that there was a significant increase in the passive stiffness of the left ventricle in heart failure with preserved ejection fraction. There is a leftward and upward shift of the diastolic pressure–volume curve indicating decreased left ventricular compliance. I bars: standard error; V: volume.

Reproduced with permission from Massachusetts Medical Society (Zile MR, Baicu CF, Gaasch WH. Diastolic heart failure-abnormalities in active relaxation and passive stiffness of the left ventricle. *N Engl J Med* 2004;350:1953–9).

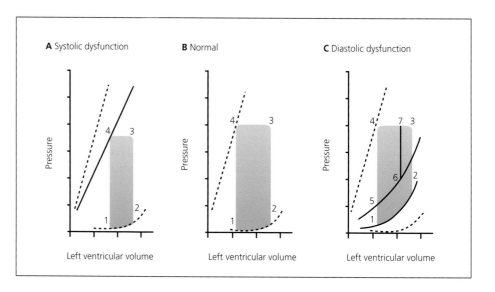

Figure 14. Schematic illustrations of left ventricular pressure–volume loops in normal individuals (B), in patients with systolic dysfunction (A), and patients with diastolic dysfunction (C). The straight dotted line is the end systolic pressure–volume relation and the curved dotted line represents the normal pressure–volume relation during diastole. The shaded area represents the pressure–volume loop area. 1 indicates opening of the mitral valve (beginning of ventricular filling), 2 the end of the filling phase, 3 the beginning of ejection, and 4 the end of ejection. The stroke volume is represented by the distance between 3 and 4. In patients with systolic dysfunction, the end systolic pressure–volume relation (straight solid line) shifts downwards and to the right due to impaired contractile function resulting in decreased stroke volume. In patients with heart failure due to diastolic dysfunction the diastolic pressure–volume relation shifts upwards and to the left (lower curved solid line), and with further increase in left ventricular stiffness the diastolic pressure–volume relation shifts further upwards and to the left (upper curved solid line). As a result the filling phase (distance between 5 and 6) is markedly reduced resulting in reduced stroke volume (distance between 7 and 4). Note that there is no shift of the straight dotted line indicating no change in contractile function.

Reproduced with permission from Elsevier Inc. (Chatterjee K, Massie B. Systolic and diastolic heart failure: differences and similarities. *J Card Fail* 2007;13:569–76).

Neurohormonal activation

Neurohormonal activation occurs in heart failure with both reduced and preserved EF, and can promote remodeling. Although the precise mechanisms responsible for activation of the neurohormonal systems remain uncertain, an increase in LV regional and global wall stress may be responsible. In patients whose heart failure is associated with reduced EF, and particularly those with CAD and MI, there is activation of vasodilatory, natriuretic, and antiproliferative agents (eg, atrial and B-type natriuretic peptides [BNPs], nitric oxide/endothelium-derived relaxing factors), as well as vasoconstrictive, antinatriuretic, proliferative, and proinflammatory agents (eg, catecholamines, angiotensins, aldosterone, endothelins, cytokines). A balance between these two systems has the potential to attenuate ventricular remodeling; an imbalance, however, can cause progressive remodeling and heart failure (**Figure 15**).

Impaired LV systolic function (reduced EF) can establish a vicious cycle of heart failure (**Figure 16**). Decreased cardiac output and LV stroke volume results in activation of

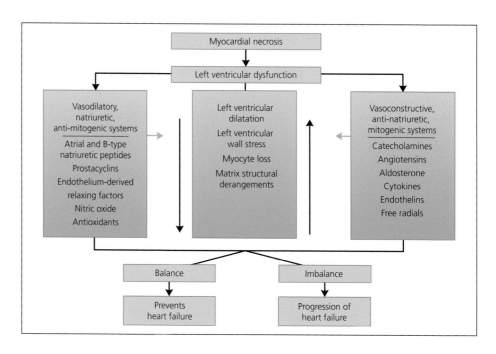

Figure 15. Neurohormonal activation following acute myocardial infarction and its contribution to left ventricular remodeling.

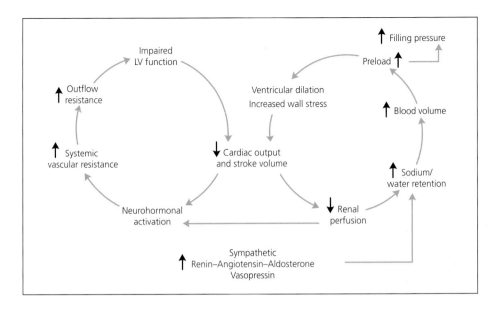

Figure 16. The vicious cycles of heart failure that may occur due to left ventricular systolic dysfunction.

the neurohormonal system, which causes an increase in systemic vascular and LV outflow resistances producing further impairment of LV systolic function. Decreased cardiac output is also associated with reduced renal perfusion, which causes increased sodium and water retention, blood volume, and preload. Increased preload not only causes an increase in LV filling pressure, but also wall stress with further impairment of systolic function.

Neurohormonal activation produces adverse ventricular and vascular remodeling, and promotes the development of atheroma (with or without thrombosis) and an inflammatory response, with further progression of remodeling and worsening heart failure.

In patients with reduced EF, neurohormonal activation occurs even without clinical heart failure; plasma norepinephrine levels, plasma renin activity, plasma vasopressin levels, and natriuretic peptide levels are all increased. In patients with clinical heart failure, levels of these neurohormones are further elevated (**Figure 17**) [11].

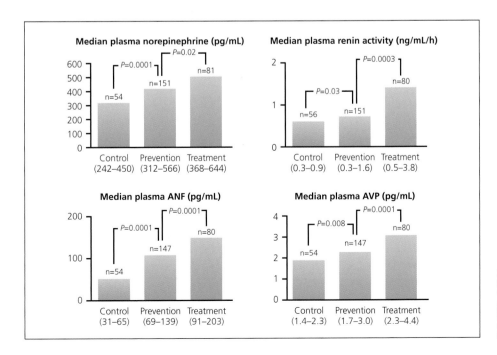

Figure 17. Neurohormonal values in patients with reduced ejection fraction with (treatment) and without (prevention) clinical heart failure compared with normal controls. ANF: atrial natriuretic factor; AVP: arginine vasopressin.

Reproduced with permission from Lippincott Williams and Wilkins (Francis GS, Benedict C, Jonstone D, et al. Comparison of neuroendocrine activation in patients with left ventricular dysfunction with and without congestive heart failure. *Circulation* 1990;82:1724–9).

CLASSIFICATION

The manner of clinical presentation of the patient determines whether he/she has acute or chronic heart failure. A sudden presentation implies acute heart failure, while a more gradual presentation suggests chronic heart failure. Patients who have had heart failure may be in a compensated or decompensated state. Once a patient has had the diagnosis of heart failure made, he remains a "case" of heart failure. However, a patient with compensated heart failure may become decompensated, a condition known as an exacerbation of heart failure.

The etiology and nature of the cardiac abnormality (eg, the various clinical syndromes of CAD that cause myocardial dysfunction, other cardiomyopathies, valve disease, congenital heart disease, pericardial disease) is also used in the classification of heart failure patients.

As the most frequent cause of heart failure is LV myocardial disease (see **Epidemiology**), a further classification of myocardial disease needs to be adopted. This classification relates to the abnormal function of the ventricle, and whether it occurs in systole or in diastole. The physiologic derangement is usually a mixture of systolic and diastolic dysfunction, one of which will often be dominant. Rather than using the phrases "systolic" and "diastolic" heart failure, however, it may be more appropriate to classify patients with myocardial disease into those with "reduced EF" and those with "preserved EF" (see **Pathophysiology**). The physiologic characteristic of EF is used because it can be readily measured by echocardiography in most patients.

It can be seen that the clinician should be able to not only determine whether the individual patient has heart failure, based on the definitions discussed at the beginning of this chapter, but also to classify heart failure patients into cases of acute heart failure, chronic heart failure, or an exacerbation of heart failure.

The clinician should indicate the etiology and nature of the underlying cardiac abnormality, and, in cases of myocardial disease, whether the patient has reduced or preserved EF.

The final challenge for the clinician is to determine the reasons for the patient presenting with heart failure at this particular time. For instance, patients with acute heart failure may present because of the development of acute MI, while patients with an exacerbation of heart failure may do so because the cardiac rhythm has changed from sinus to atrial fibrillation. This is discussed in further detail in the next section.

PRESENTATION

Acute heart failure

Patients with acute heart failure are usually extremely ill. They present with acute breathlessness and impaired perfusion to the vital organs. Breathlessness is mainly caused by pulmonary congestion due to increased pulmonary venous pressure, usually due to a rise in LV filling pressure. Lying flat increases pulmonary venous pressure further and causes orthopnea; this may progress to the development of frank pulmonary edema, causing attacks of paroxysmal nocturnal dyspnea. A cough productive of pink, frothy sputum is characteristic. Pulmonary edema is often incorrectly diagnosed as bronchitis.

An acute reduction in cardiac output leads to impaired perfusion of vital organs. Thus, impaired cerebral perfusion may result in an altered level of consciousness, while impaired renal perfusion may result in oliguria.

Auscultation of the lungs reveals bilateral crackles. Cardiogenic shock might be present, with low blood pressure, tachycardia, and peripheral vasoconstriction. Other features might include pulsus alternans (**Figure 18**) and an elevated jugular venous pressure (**Figure 1**). Peripheral edema will not be present.

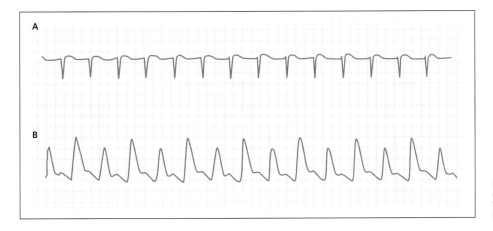

Figure 18. An arterial pulse tracing (B) with a simultaneous electrocardiogram (A) in a patient with heart failure and reduced ejection fraction. The arterial pulse tracing shows alternating weaker and stronger pulses (pulsus alternans).

Physical signs in the heart (which can be difficult to elicit because the patient is seriously ill) may reflect the underlying cardiac abnormality responsible for the development of acute heart failure. Thus, in patients in whom the underlying abnormality is LV myocardial dysfunction, a third heart sound (S3) or gallop rhythm (the summation of a third and fourth [S4] heart sound in the presence of a sinus tachycardia resulting in a short diastole [**Figure 2**]) may be heard. These additional heart sounds correlate with abnormal hemodynamic findings in such patients, notably a raised LV end-diastolic pressure. A pansystolic murmur might be heard; this can be due to mitral regurgitation secondary to LV dysfunction, or because there is acute severe primary mitral regurgitation as a result of chordal rupture in patients who have "floppy" mitral valves (**Figure 19**). Because a frequent precipitating factor for the development of acute heart failure is the sudden development of atrial fibrillation, this rhythm may be present on examination.

If the underlying cardiac abnormality is not LV dysfunction the patient's physical signs can reveal the nature of the abnormality. For example, aortic stenosis is characterized by a slow-rising arterial pulse, while mitral stenosis is indicated by an opening snap and a mid-diastolic murmur on auscultation.

Chronic heart failure

The patient with chronic heart failure presents in a more insidious way. The most frequent symptom is progressive breathlessness. Initially, the patient may only notice breathlessness on exertion, but the degree of exertion that brings on the breathlessness gradually becomes less and less. Eventually, the patient may notice breathlessness on trivial exertion or even at rest, often with an accompanying cough.

The mechanism of breathlessness in chronic heart failure is complex. An imbalance in ventilation and perfusion in the lungs is thought to be the most important factor, but impaired diaphragmatic function and skeletal muscle ergoreflexes may contribute to exaggerated ventilatory responses and the sensation of breathlessness. The muscle

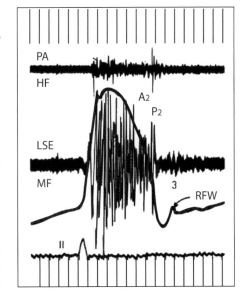

Figure 19. Simultaneous phonocardiograms in the pulmonary area (PA) recorded using high frequency filters (HF) and at the left sternal edge (LSE) using medium frequency filters (MF), lead II of the electrocardiogram, together with an apex cardiogram in a patient with mitral regurgitation due to ruptured chordae tendineae. A pansystolic murmur is recorded at the LSE, and there is also a third heart sound (3) corresponding with the peak of the rapid filling wave (RFW) in the apex cardiogram. The two components of the second heart sound (aortic valve closure [A2] and pulmonary valve closure [P2]) are seen in the phonocardiograms.

ergoreflex systems are located in the exercising muscles, and the afferent pathways are activated during exercise. This is quite different to the mechanism in acute heart failure, where the dominant influence is the rise in pulmonary venous pressure.

Fatigue is a common symptom in patients with chronic heart failure. This probably relates to inadequate blood flow to exercising muscle. Patients with chronic heart failure may notice fluid retention, with swollen ankles and abdominal distention due to ascites and/or hepatic congestion. These features probably develop as a result of stimulation of the renin–angiotensin–aldosterone system. The patient with chronic heart failure may complain of nausea, vomiting, and abdominal discomfort due to gastrointestinal and hepatic congestion; such patients are frequently thought to have abdominal pathology rather than heart failure.

Other symptoms in patients with chronic heart failure relate to the underlying cardiac pathology responsible for the development of heart failure. Thus, patients who have LV dysfunction secondary to CAD may experience angina, patients with aortic stenosis may experience exertional syncope, and patients with established atrial fibrillation may experience palpitation.

Abnormal physical signs in the patient with chronic heart failure include an elevated jugular venous pressure (**Figure 1**), hepatojugular reflux (**Figure 20**), edema of the ankles, legs, and sacrum, an enlarged liver, and even ascites (**Figures 21** and **22**). These findings reflect the fluid retention that is characteristic of decompensated chronic heart failure.

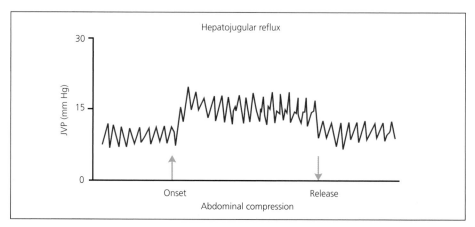

Figure 20. A schematic illustration of a positive hepato-jugular (hepato-abdominal) reflux in a patient with heart failure and reduced ejection fraction. The changes in jugular venous pressure (JVP) during abdominal compression are illustrated. With the onset of compression, JVP increases substantially and remains elevated for as long as the compression is maintained.

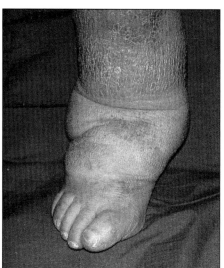
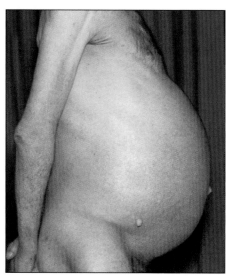

Figure 21 (left). Severe ankle edema in a patient with chronic heart failure.

Figure 22 (right). Severe abdominal distension due to hepatic distension and ascites in a patient with chronic heart failure.

Other physical signs may indicate whether the heart failure is due to myocardial dysfunction or to some other cardiac abnormality. Myocardial diastolic dysfunction renders the ventricles stiff, augmenting atrial contraction in an attempt to deliver blood into the stiff ventricle. This enhanced atrial contraction (which can be auscultated as the fourth heart sound [S4]) can also be palpated separately from the normal outward movement during ventricular systole. Palpation of the two outward movements, one during atrial systole and the other during ventricular systole, results in a "double" apical impulse (**Figure 23**). A sustained outward movement is another characteristic of the cardiac impulse. Usually this is characteristic of a pressure-loaded ventricle (as in aortic stenosis), but it can also occur in a dilated left ventricle with reduced EF and stroke volume. A third heart sound (S3) may also be heard. If sinus tachycardia is present a gallop rhythm may be heard. In addition, a pansystolic murmur due to secondary mitral or tricuspid regurgitation may be present.

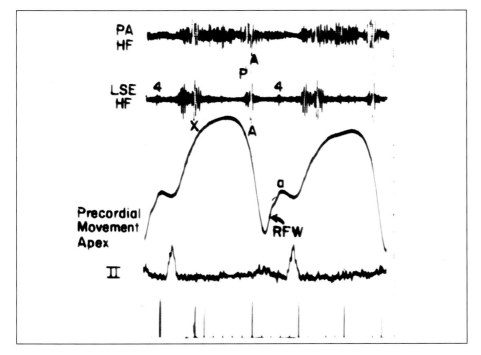

Figure 23. Simultaneous phonocardiograms recorded using high frequency filters in the pulmonary area (PA-HF) and at the left sternal edge (LSE-HF) with an apex cardiogram (precordial movement apex) and lead II of the electrocardiogram in a patient with aortic stenosis. There is a double impulse shown in the apex cardiogram, the first part of which is due to an exaggerated atrial contraction ('a' wave) immediately following the rapid filling wave (RFW), and the second part due to sustained outward movement during ventricular systole. The 'a' wave coincides with a fourth heart sound (4). An ejection sound (X) and ejection systolic murmur are seen in the phonocardiograms. Aortic valve closure (A) follows pulmonary valve closure (P) resulting in reversed splitting of the second heart sound.

Atrial fibrillation is a common finding in patients with chronic heart failure (**Figure 24**). Primary valvular abnormalities, congenital cardiac abnormalities, or pericardial disease each have their own distinctive physical signs.

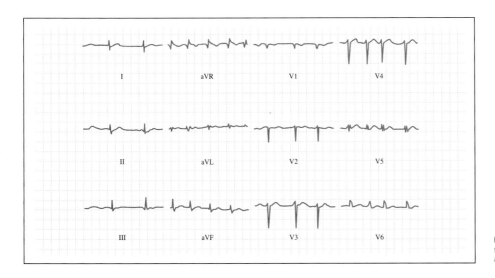

Figure 24. Electrocardiogram of a patient with dilated cardiomyopathy showing atrial fibrillation, poor R wave progression in the precordial leads, and incomplete left bundle branch block.

Exacerbation of heart failure

A patient who has had heart failure in the past may remain well compensated over long periods of time. Usually, the patient remains compensated as a result of being treated with a variety of pharmacologic agents (see **Management**). This implies that the patient can lead his/her usual life without noticing breathlessness or fatigue, or only to a minor extent. However, such a patient may deteriorate, with increasing breathlessness and fatigue, either gradually or (sometimes) abruptly. This situation is known as an exacerbation of heart failure.

Several factors are known to cause exacerbations of heart failure. A change in cardiac rhythm, when the patient was previously in sinus rhythm, is a common precipitating factor for both the development of acute heart failure and for an exacerbation of heart failure. By far the most common change in rhythm is the development of atrial fibrillation. If atrial systole is lost (as in atrial fibrillation), stroke volume and cardiac output fall, particularly in patients with preserved EF, and heart failure results. In patients with a dilated left ventricle and reduced EF, the LV stroke volume is slightly reduced when atrial systole is lost (**Figure 25**). Irrespective of the state of the EF, worsening heart failure with the development of atrial fibrillation is also due to the uncontrolled rapid ventricular rate and consequent reduction in LV filling time. This not only reduces LV stroke volume, but also increases LV diastolic pressure.

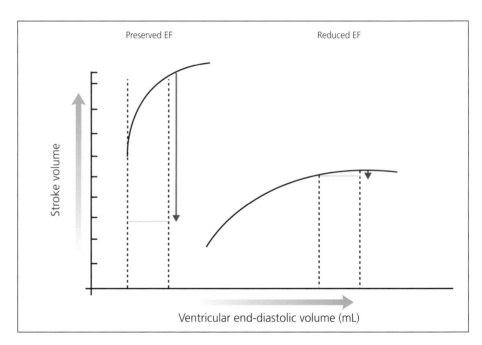

Figure 25. Differences in the magnitude of stroke volume reduction in heart failure with preserved and reduced ejection fraction, with loss of timed atrial contraction. In patients with preserved ejection fraction the left ventricular function curve is normal; with the loss of atrial contraction (atrial fibrillation) and with the reduction of end-diastolic volume there is a substantial reduction in stroke volume. In patients with reduced ejection fraction, the ventricular function curve is shifted downwards and to the right and patients with severe heart failure are represented by the flat portion of the curve with already increased end-diastolic volume. This figure demonstrates that for a particular reduction in end-diastolic volume, the corresponding stroke volume reduction is much smaller in patients with reduced ejection fraction and loss of atrial contraction (atrial fibrillation) compared with patients with preserved ejection fraction (see red arrows).

In patients who have heart failure due to CAD, the sudden development of myocardial ischemia or MI can result in a significant deterioration in LV function. If this occurs, previously compensated heart failure can become decompensated.

A common reason for patients with compensated heart failure to become more breathless and develop fluid retention with resultant weight gain is a reduction in diuretic therapy. Maintaining a balance between the retention of fluid and dehydration is a common problem in patients with chronic heart failure. Either the patient or his physician may decide to reduce the diuretic dosage, which can lead to an exacerbation of heart failure.

Chronic renal failure associated with heart failure (cardiorenal syndrome) can contribute to decompensation. Anemia, whether dilutional or due to suppression of erythropoiesis, can also cause decompensation. Uncontrolled hypertension, generalized noncardiac infection, and pulmonary embolism are other uncommon precipitating factors that may cause exacerbation of heart failure (**Table 4**).

Table 4. Factors precipitating or causing an exacerbation of heart failure [5].
Cardiac rhythm changes (particularly atrial fibrillation)
Acute myocardial infarction/ischemia
Change in therapy (particularly diuretics)
Generalized infection, uncontrolled hypertension, anemia, renal failure, pulmonary embolism all less common

INVESTIGATIONS

Investigation of the patient with heart failure is essential for an accurate diagnosis. Investigations not only provide information that helps to support the diagnosis of heart failure, but can also reveal the underlying etiology and nature of the cardiac pathology responsible for the development of heart failure. The value of the investigations relevant to the different categories of heart failure forms the basis of this section.

Acute heart failure
Plain chest X-ray
The plain chest X-ray is essential to support the diagnosis of acute heart failure. Acute heart failure usually means the development of acute pulmonary edema, which can be detected by the chest X-ray. The classical appearance of pulmonary edema is bilateral shadowing radiating from the hila ("bat's wing appearance") (**Figure 26**). This is sometimes accompanied by unilateral or bilateral pleural effusions. It is not usually possible to detect changes in the pulmonary veins reflecting the rise in pulmonary venous pressure because the hilar shadowing obscures them. The cardiothoracic ratio may be normal in acute heart failure, but it can also be increased (enlarged heart) if there is pre-existing pathology that led to the development of acute heart failure.

Resting electrocardiogram
The resting ECG does not reflect the presence of acute heart failure, but it can provide information as to the cause. A normal ECG is extremely uncommon in acute heart failure. Indeed, the negative predictive value of a normal ECG in heart failure with reduced EF exceeds 90% [12]. In acute heart failure, the rhythm may be atrial fibrillation. The ECG may show evidence of either acute MI (**Figure 27**) or acute myocardial ischemia, conditions that could have precipitated the development of acute heart failure. Other specific conditions, such as acute pericardial disease or acute myocarditis causing acute heart failure, can also produce characteristic features on the ECG (**Figure 28**).

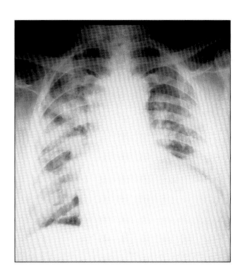

Figure 26. Chest X-ray showing cardiomegaly with bilateral shadowing in the lungs characteristic of pulmonary edema.

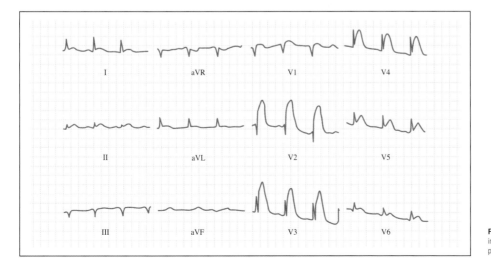

Figure 27. Electrocardiogram showing early changes of anterior myocardial infarction. There is ST-segment elevation in leads I and II, and in the precordial leads, but without Q waves.

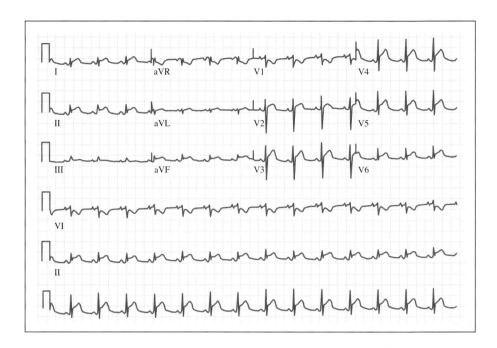

Figure 28. Electrocardiogram showing generalized ST-segment elevation consistent with acute pericarditis.

B-type natriuretic peptide

BNP is elevated in patients with acute heart failure or an exacerbation of chronic heart failure. A normal BNP level excludes breathlessness of cardiac origin (**Figure 29**) [13].

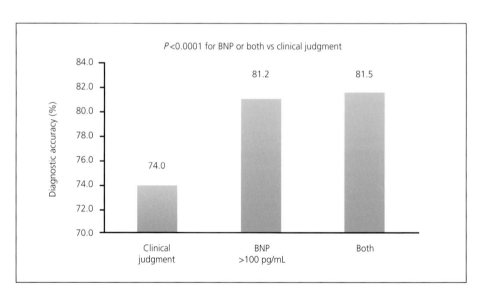

Figure 29. Value of B-type natriuretic peptide (BNP) levels for the diagnosis of acute dyspnea of cardiac origin in patients presenting in the emergency department. The diagnostic accuracy of the clinical judgment of the attending physicians was 74%. If the BNP level was >100 pg/mL, the diagnostic accuracy was 81.2%; the diagnostic accuracy of combined abnormal BNP level and clinical judgment was the same at 81.5%.

Reproduced with permission from Lippincott Williams and Wilkins (McCullough PA, Nowak RM, McCord J, et al. B-type natriuretic peptide and clinical judgment in the emergency diagnosis of heart failure: analysis from the Breathing Not Properly (BNP) Multinational Study. *Circulation* 2002;106:416–22).

Chronic heart failure

Plain chest X-ray

The plain chest X-ray of chronic heart failure contrasts with that of acute heart failure. An enlarged heart (increased cardiothoracic ratio) implies pre-existing heart disease. In chronic heart failure, the heart is usually enlarged and there might be radiographic features associated with raised pulmonary venous pressure (**Figures 30** and **31**). These include dilatation of the upper zone pulmonary vessels and left atrial enlargement (**Figure 32**), Kerley B-lines (short horizontal lines in the peripheral lung fields) (**Figure 33**), and, occasionally, unilateral or bilateral pleural effusions (**Figure 34**). These abnormal radiographic appearances correlate with the elevation of LV diastolic, left atrial, and pulmonary venous pressures. It should be emphasized that the chest X-ray findings are the same in patients with reduced or preserved EF.

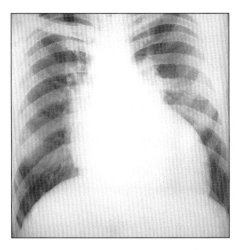

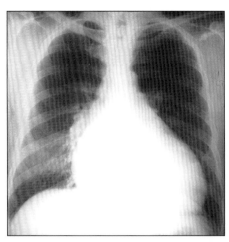

Figure 30 (left). Chest X-ray showing cardiomegaly with upper zone blood diversion.

Figure 31 (right). Chest X-ray showing cardiomegaly without upper zone blood diversion.

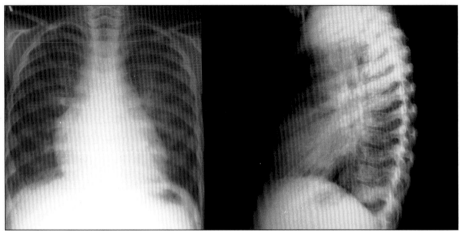

Figure 32. Chest X-ray (posteroanterior and left lateral projections) showing left atrial enlargement with dilatation of the upper zone pulmonary vessels.

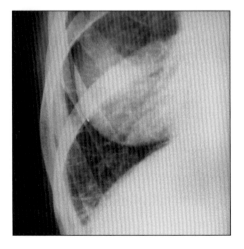

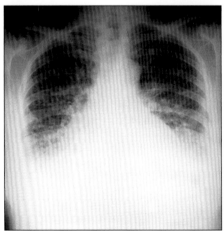

Figure 33 (left). Detail from chest X-ray showing septal lines (Kerley B-lines) and pleural effusion.

Figure 34 (right). Chest X-ray showing bilateral pleural effusions.

Resting electrocardiogram

The ECG in chronic heart failure may show evidence of a previous MI or extensive damage to the left ventricle as a result of CAD. Thus, there may be pathologic Q-waves, an arborization type of left bundle branch block, or persistent Q-waves and ST segment elevation characteristic of an LV aneurysm (**Figures 35–37**). The ECG may also show evidence of LV hypertrophy, left atrial enlargement, or nonspecific ST-T changes (**Figures 38** and **39**). Approximately 30% of patients with advanced heart failure develop atrial fibrillation (**Figure 24**), irrespective of whether EF is reduced or preserved. In general the ECG does not distinguish between heart failure with reduced or preserved EF.

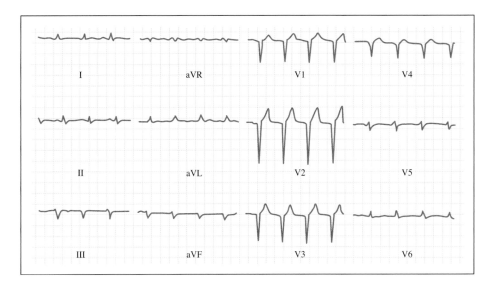

Figure 35. Electrocardiogram from a patient with ischemic heart disease showing old anterior myocardial infarction with Q-waves in V1–V4 and poor R-wave progression in V5–V6.

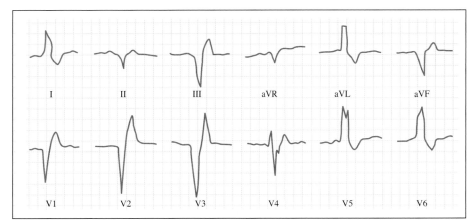

Figure 36. Electrocardiogram from a patient with dilated cardiomyopathy showing left bundle branch block.

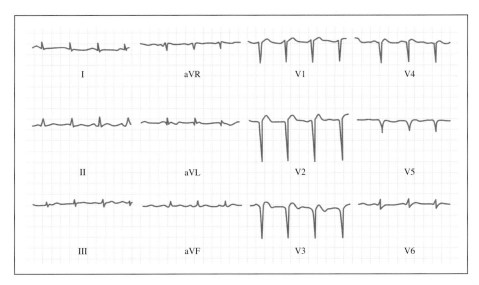

Figure 37. Electrocardiogram from a patient with a left ventricular aneurysm showing Q-waves and ST segment elevation in the anterior chest leads 6 months after myocardial infarction.

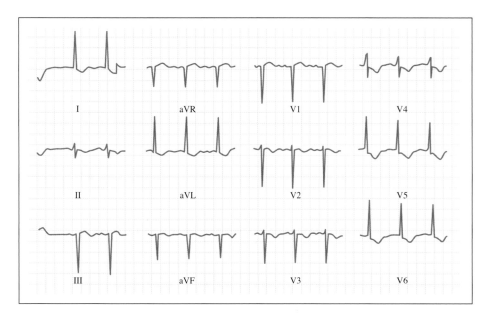

Figure 38. Electrocardiogram showing both increased voltage and ST-T abnormalities consistent with left ventricular hypertrophy.

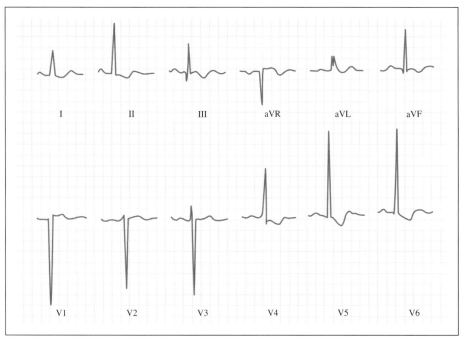

Figure 39. Electrocardiogram from a patient with dilated cardiomyopathy showing nonspecific ST-T abnormalities.

Natriuretic peptides

A number of biomarkers have been investigated as aids to the diagnosis of heart failure. Of these, the natriuretic peptides have emerged as the most useful in making and, particularly, excluding the diagnosis of heart failure.

In patients with heart failure natriuretic peptides are synthesized and released from both ventricles and atria in response to wall stress, whether it results from pressure or volume overload. BNP is primarily synthesized and released by ventricular myocytes, although it was originally identified in porcine brain (hence its name).

Atrial natriuretic peptides, BNP, N-terminal BNP, urodilatin, and other natriuretic peptides have all been investigated. Of these, BNP has been found to be the most useful in differentiating between breathlessness due to a cardiac or noncardiac cause (**Figure 40**) [14].

Figure 40. Value of B-type natriuretic peptide (BNP) levels in the differential diagnosis of cardiac and noncardiac dyspnea. In patients without heart failure the BNP level is usually <100 pg/mL. In patients who have left ventricular dysfunction, but whose dyspnea is due to noncardiac causes, the BNP level is only modestly increased. In patients with overt heart failure, it is markedly elevated.

Reproduced with permission from Massachusetts Medical Society (Maisel AS, Krishnaswamy P, Nowak RM, et al. Rapid measurement of B-type natriuretic peptide in the emergency diagnosis of heart failure. *N Engl J Med* 2002;347:161–7). .

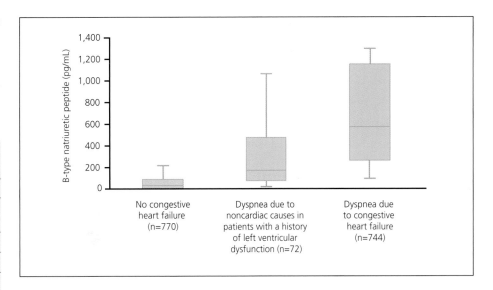

Table 5. Conditions in which B-type natriuretic peptide levels can be raised.
Acute heart failure
Chronic heart failure (reduced or preserved ejection fraction)
Cor pulmonale, acute or chronic
Acute coronary syndromes
Stable angina
Asymptomatic left ventricular systolic dysfunction
Valvular heart disease
Atrial fibrillation
Ventricular hypertrophy
Isolated atrial enlargement
Renal failure
(NB. B-type natriuretic peptide levels can be decreased in obesity)

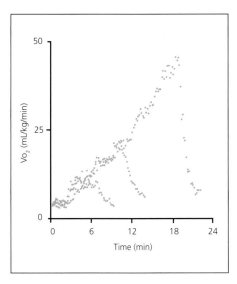

Figure 41. Oxygen consumption (VO₂) during symptom-limited treadmill exercise and on recovery, in a normal patient (right), a patient with moderate heart failure (middle) and a patient with severe heart failure (left). At rest and during the first 5 minutes of exercise all three subjects have similar oxygen consumption, but peak VO₂ is progressively reduced as the severity of heart failure increases

In patients who present with breathlessness, whether during physical activity or at rest, a BNP level of <100 pg/mL virtually excludes the possibility of a cardiac origin. An exception to this rule is the obese patient with a high body mass index, in whom BNP levels can be surprisingly low despite obvious heart failure. This is probably due to overexpression of natriuretic peptide clearance receptors in the adipocytes. It should also be recognized that an elevated BNP level can be found in many conditions, with or without clinically evident heart failure (**Table 5**).

Exercise testing

Exercise testing is frequently performed to assess functional impairment in chronic heart failure. A 6-minute walk distance measurement is often carried out. Maximal or submaximal tests on a treadmill or bicycle ergometer, with measurement of exercise time, may also be performed (**Figure 41**). Maximal oxygen consumption (VO₂ max) can be used to assess the severity of heart failure. In patients with no or mild heart failure VO₂ is >20 mL/kg/min, while in severe heart failure VO₂ is usually ≤6 mL/kg/min. When VO₂ max is <14 mL/kg/min the prognosis is grave and the VO₂ max level is used as an indication for cardiac transplantation.

Exacerbation of heart failure

If a patient in a steady state of heart failure deteriorates, the presentation can be either acute or insidious. For the relevant investigations in patients who deteriorate acutely, see those described under "acute heart failure"; for patients who present insidiously, see the "chronic heart failure" section.

Etiology of heart failure
Echocardiography and Doppler

Echocardiography is the most frequently used investigation to establish the cause of heart failure. The echocardiographic features will reflect the underlying cardiac abnormality. In patients with CAD there may be an increase in LV dimensions and a reduction in wall motion, which can be regional (**Figure 42**) or generalized. A global reduction in the amplitude of wall motion is more frequent in idiopathic dilated cardiomyopathy (**Figure 43**). These appearances are seen in LV myocardial disease with reduced EF.

The appearance of the left ventricle in either extensive CAD or idiopathic dilated cardiomyopathy is frequently difficult to assess. This is due to the presence of left bundle

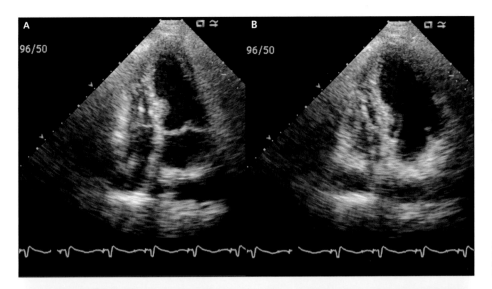

Figure 42. Apical four-chamber views at end-systole (A) and end-diastole (B). At end-diastole (B), the mid to distal septum appears thinned and slightly aneurysmal, indicating probable infarction. The end-systolic image (A) shows an apical wall motion abnormality.

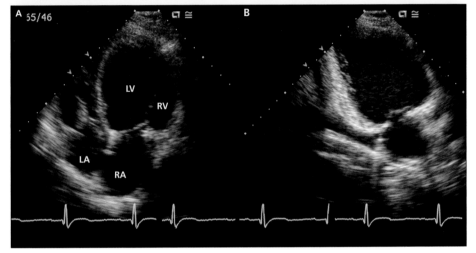

Figure 43. Apical four-chamber view (A) and two-chamber view (B) showing a markedly enlarged and spherical left ventricle (LV). LA: left atrium; RA: right atrium; RV: right ventricle.

branch block, which in itself causes dyskinetic contraction. Systolic wall thinning and/or dyskinesia are readily apparent from inspection of the systolic and diastolic images. Dyskinesia should not be confused with dyssynchrony, which reflects abnormal contraction and relaxation of the segments of the ventricular wall. Enlargement of the left atrium due to chronic elevation of the LV filling pressure is common (**Figure 44**).

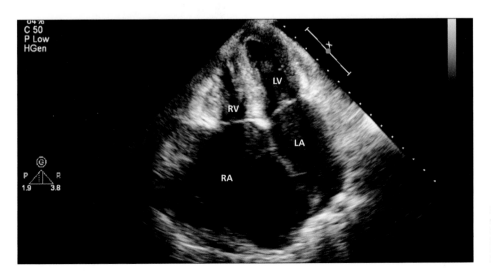

Figure 44. Apical four-chamber view showing normal ventricular volumes with marked biatrial enlargement, including the left atrium, in a patient with restrictive cardiomyopathy and chronic increase in left ventricular diastolic pressure. The right atrium is also markedly enlarged due to pulmonary hypertension and tricuspid regurgitation. LA: left atrium; LV: left ventricle; RA: right atrium; RV: right ventricle.

Doppler echocardiography is useful in excluding primary valvular heart disease as the cause of heart failure. The Doppler technique may reveal mitral regurgitation of varying severity secondary to LV myocardial disease (**Figure 45**).

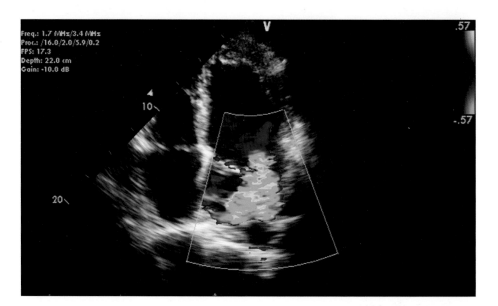

Figure 45. Apical four-chamber view. Color flow Doppler demonstrates a wide jet of mitral regurgitation (light blue and yellow) occupying >50% of the left atrium.

Doppler transmitral flow patterns in patients with heart failure in sinus rhythm are variable. In the early stages, impaired relaxation leads to decreased amplitude and prolonged duration of the early filling ("E") wave with a compensatory increase in the atrial filling ("A") wave, resulting in a decreased E:A ratio (**Figure 46**). In the late stages, an accentuated E-wave amplitude and reduced A-wave amplitude, implying a restrictive physiology, may be seen (**Figure 47**). In dilated cardiomyopathy, an abbreviated E-wave with decreased deceleration time and reduced A-wave amplitude are associated with a poor prognosis. In patients whose heart failure is due to dominant diastolic dysfunction (as in systemic hypertension), the E-wave is decreased and the A-wave accentuated, while the left ventricle is seen to be hypertrophied but contracts normally (**Figure 48**). In patients with heart failure with preserved EF, an accentuated A-wave with a decreased E-wave, or a normal or even restrictive pattern, can be seen.

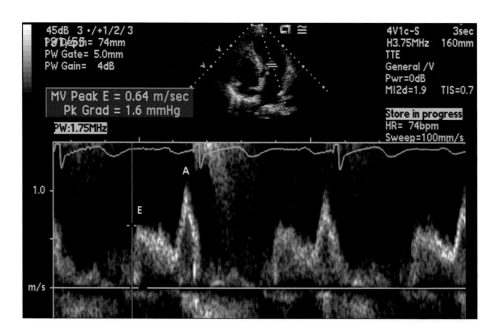

Figure 46. Pulsed wave Doppler of mitral inflow demonstrating a higher "A" wave velocity than "E" wave velocity, consistent with impaired left ventricular relaxation. A: flow during atrial contraction; E: early filling wave.

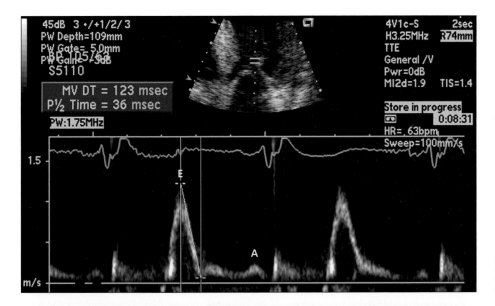

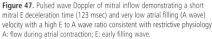

Figure 47. Pulsed wave Doppler of mitral inflow demonstrating a short mitral E deceleration time (123 msec) and very low atrial filling (A wave) velocity with a high E to A wave ratio consistent with restrictive physiology. A: flow during atrial contraction; E: early filling wave.

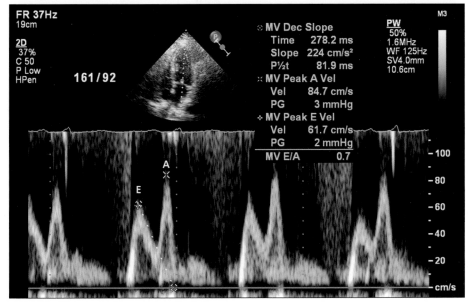

Figure 48. Pulsed wave Doppler of mitral inflow demonstrating an increase in "A" wave velocity in a patient with hypertensive heart disease. A: flow during atrial contraction; E: early filling wave.

The presence of tricuspid regurgitation in patients with heart failure allows noninvasive measurement of the pulmonary artery systolic pressure (**Figures 49** and **50**). If tricuspid regurgitation is primary, or secondary due to pulmonary hypertension, the right ventricle is dilated. The pulmonary artery systolic pressure is only slightly elevated in patients with LV disease, in contrast to the severe elevation of pulmonary artery systolic pressure in cases of long-standing pulmonary hypertension. In patients with heart failure due to severe pulmonary hypertension, but without left heart disease, there may be paradoxical septal motion and right ventricular hypertrophy and dilatation (**Figure 51**).

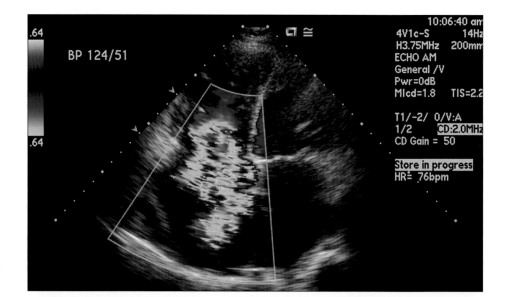

Figure 49 (right). Color flow Doppler across the tricuspid valve showing a large jet of severe tricuspid regurgitation. The right atrium and ventricle are enlarged.

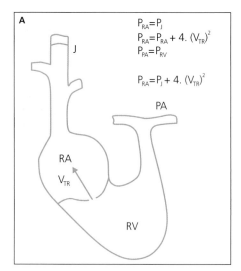

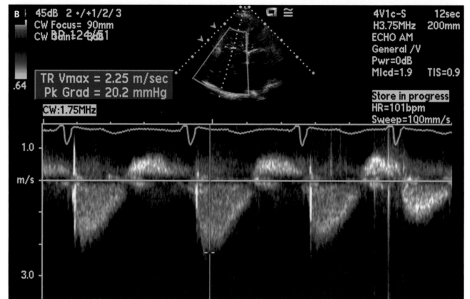

Figure 50. (A) Diagram showing the basis for assessment of pulmonary hypertension using continuous-wave spectral Doppler. Pressure in the right atrium (P_{RA}) can be determined from inspection of the jugular venous pulse. If any tricuspid regurgitation is present, the Bernoulli equation ($\Delta P=4xV^2$) allows the (RV–RA) pressure gradient to be calculated from the velocity of the jet (V_{TR}). Systolic pressure in the right ventricle (P_{RV}) equals that in the pulmonary arteries (P_{PA}) as long as there is no right ventricular outflow obstruction. (B) Continuous-wave spectral Doppler of tricuspid regurgitation. The peak jet velocity is 2.25 m/s, corresponding to an RV–RA gradient of 20.2 mm Hg. Pulmonary artery pressure is thus equal to RA pressure +20.2 mm Hg. J: jugular vein; PA: pulmonary arteries; RA: right atrium; RV: right ventricle.

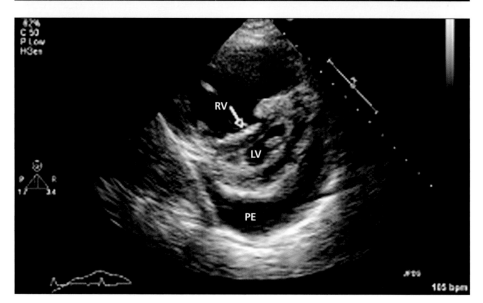

Figure 51. An echocardiogram of a patient with severe pulmonary arterial hypertension showing a dilated right ventricle (RV) and a shift of the septum (arrow), reducing the size of the left ventricle (LV). Pericardial effusion (PE) is also present.

Nuclear techniques

When it is impossible to assess the function of the left ventricle by echocardiography, an alternative technique is to perform radionuclide ventriculography using technetium-99m to label the intracardiac blood pool. Usually imaging is performed during the equilibrium phase (**Figure 52**) [15]. LV volumes, EF, and parameters of diastolic function, such as filling rates, can be measured (**Figure 53**) [16]. Using this technique, it is possible to classify patients with heart failure into those who have reduced EF and those who have preserved EF. Right ventricular systolic function can also be assessed.

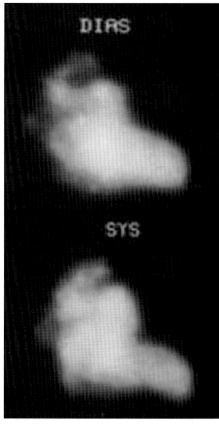

Figure 52 (above). Assessment of left ventricular function by single photon emission computed tomography blood pool imaging using the equilibrium technique. In a patient with heart failure and reduced ejection fraction there is left ventricular enlargement in both end diastole (DIAS) and in end systole (SYS), together with apical akinesis.

Reproduced with permission from FA Davis Company (Botvinick EH, Glazer H, Shosa D. What is the reliability and utility of scintigraphic methods for the assessment of ventricular function? *Cardiovascular Clin* 1983;13:65–78).

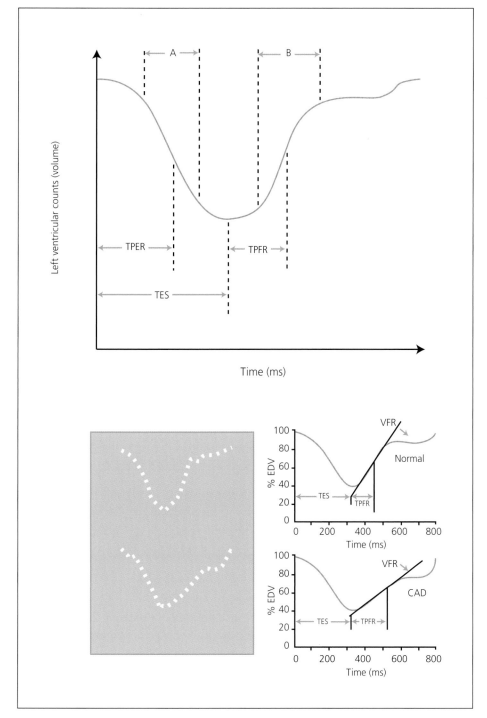

Figure 53. Filling phase indices. The upper panel shows a diagrammatic left ventricular radioactivity (counts) versus time curve indicating time to peak emptying rate (TPER), time to peak filling rate (TPFR), and time to end systole (TES) during systolic (A) and diastolic (B) periods. In the lower panel, actual curves and diagrammatic representations are shown in a normal individual (top) and in a patient with coronary artery disease (CAD, bottom) revealing a reduced ventricular filling rate (VFR).
EDV: end-diastolic filling volume.

Reproduced with permission from Lippincott Williams and Wilkins (Bonow RR, Bacharach SL, Green MV, et al. Impaired left ventricular diastolic filling in patients with coronary artery disease. Assessment with radionuclide angiography. *Circulation* 1981;64:315–23).

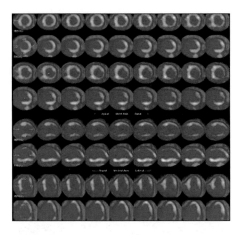

Figure 54 (above). Gated perfusion single photon emission computed tomography dual isotope imaging using thallium-201 (rest, even rows)/technicium-99m sestamibi (stress-related, odd rows) to detect the presence and extent of ischemic myocardium. The first 4 rows (from top) show short axis slices from apex (left) to base (right). Rows 5 and 6 show vertical long axis slices from septum (left) to lateral wall (right) and rows 7 and 8 show horizontal long axis slices from inferior wall (left) to anterior wall (right). A large reversible perfusion defect in the antero-lateral wall of the left ventricle (distribution of the left anterior descending coronary artery territory) is evident, indicating the presence of ischemic myocardium.

Courtesy of E. Botvinick, University of California, San Francisco.

Figure 55 (right). Radionuclide (scintigraphic) evaluation of the presence and extent of viable ischemic myocardium by positron emission tomography. Short axis slices (rows 1–4), vertical long axis slices (rows 5 and 6), and horizontal long axis slices (rows 7 and 8) are shown. The resting perfusion images with rubidium-82 (rows 1, 3, 5, and 7) demonstrate a large lateral wall perfusion defect, but other areas take up rubidium-82 indicating that these are perfused and viable. The fluor-deoxyglucose images (rows 2, 4, 6, and 8) reveal complementary uptake, which indicates active myocardial metabolism and thus myocardial viability.

Courtesy of E. Botvinick, University of California, San Francisco.

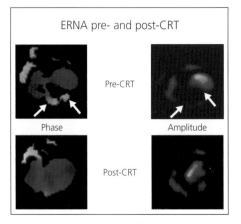

Figure 56 (above). Phase image analysis of left ventricular synchrony before (top) and after (bottom) cardiac resynchronization treatment (CRT). Phase (left) and amplitude images (right) are derived from gated equilibrium radionuclide angiograms (ERNAs) in a patient with heart failure and reduced ejection fraction. Pre-CRT images show severe regional dyssynchrony in the phase image (white arrows) involving the septum and the apex. There is reduced amplitude in most of the distal left ventricle as shown by the low intensity regions in the same areas (white arrows) of the amplitude image. In the post-CRT images, color and phase are more synchronous, with much improvement in intensity of the amplitude image, indicating improved systolic motion following CRT.

Courtesy of E. Botvinick, University of California, San Francisco.

Thallium-201 imaging is a technique that investigates the cause of heart failure; it can reveal extensive myocardial ischemia as a result of CAD. Significant thallium uptake in areas of wall motion abnormality suggests "hibernation" (**Figure 54**). Hibernation indicates impaired, but reversible, regional myocardial systolic function as a result of chronic ischemia of the myocardium. Following reperfusion of these ischemic segments the function of the myocardium improves due to an improvement in regional wall motion. If significant reversible myocardial perfusion defects are detected, coronary arteriography is indicated. Entirely normal myocardial perfusion images virtually exclude CAD as the cause of heart failure. Myocardial perfusion and metabolism can be assessed by positron emission tomography to enable a diagnosis of hibernating myocardium to be made (**Figure 55**). Radionuclide ventriculography is employed to detect LV dyssynchrony before cardiac resynchronization therapy (CRT) is undertaken. It is also used to determine the result of such treatment on synchronization (**Figure 56**).

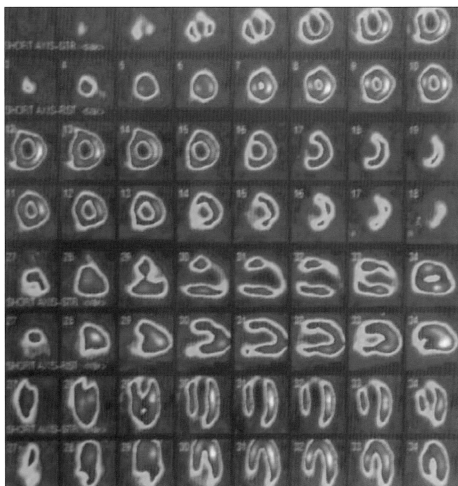

Magnetic resonance imaging and computed tomography

MRI and CT noninvasively reveal cardiac anatomy, with or without the injection of contrast media. Accurate measurements of ventricular volumes (**Figure 57**) and wall thickness can be made, and wall motion assessed (**Figure 58**). Filling defects such as thrombus are readily detected. Both MRI and CT are useful in excluding pericardial disease. The delayed/enhancement MRI technique is also used for the diagnosis of myocarditis. This technique provides MRI images that are acquired in end-diastole 20–30 minutes after a bolus injection of gadolinium (a contrast medium). Persistent hyperenhancement is present if there is an inflamed area of myocardium.

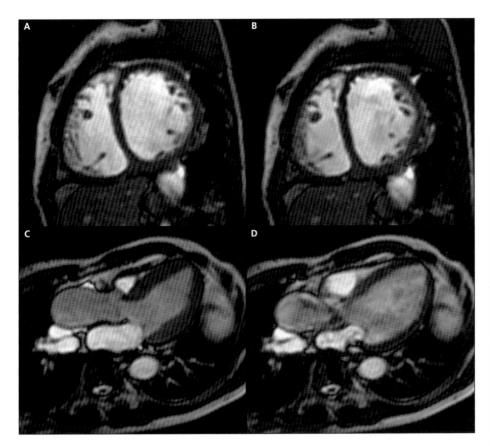

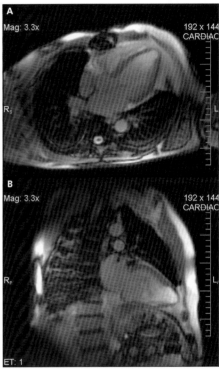

Figure 57 (left). Cardiac magnetic resonance imaging with contrast injection to assess left ventricular volumes. End-systolic frames (A and C) and end-diastolic frames (B and D) are shown in lateral (top) and anterior oblique (bottom) views, respectively. In the lateral views both right and left ventricular images are shown. In the anterior oblique views only the left ventricle is shown.

Courtesy of G. Reddy, University of California, San Francisco.

Figure 58 (above). Cardiac magnetic resonance imaging (anterior oblique view [A] and lateral view [B]) to assess left ventricular wall motion abnormalities. A shows an end-diastolic frame and B shows an end-systolic frame in a patient with dilated cardiomyopathy. There is very little change in left ventricular diameters, which are generally hypokinetic.

Courtesy of G. Reddy, University of California, San Francisco.

Cardiac catheterization and coronary arteriography

Bedside monitoring of right heart pressures is occasionally useful in the differential diagnosis of patients with acute heart failure. A multipurpose balloon-tipped thermodilution, electrode, and multiporous catheter, positioned with its tip in the pulmonary artery, allows accurate measurement of pulmonary artery and wedge pressures and cardiac output (**Figure 59**). This measurement may facilitate the assessment of the severity of the hemodynamic abnormalities and the results of therapeutic interventions. In addition, temporary cardiac pacing can be performed and the infusion channels can be used for intravenous (IV) drug infusion.

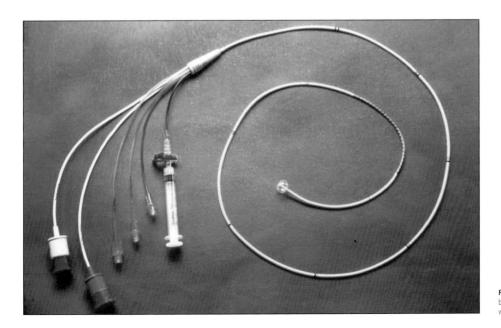

Figure 59. A multipurpose thermodilution, electrode, and multiporous balloon flotation catheter, which can be inserted at the bedside without fluoroscopy.

The hemodynamic changes in patients with heart failure are variable. In symptomatic patients, elevated LV diastolic, left atrial, and pulmonary venous pressures are almost invariably present. In patients with advanced heart failure, pulmonary hypertension with secondary tricuspid regurgitation and elevation of the right atrial pressure with a dominant V-wave are present, irrespective of whether the heart failure is due to myocardial dysfunction with reduced or preserved EF.

In the early stages of heart failure cardiac output is usually normal at rest, but it may not increase appropriately during exercise. In patients with advanced heart failure, cardiac output may be decreased even at rest. Relative hypotension due to decreased stroke volume and impaired organ perfusion (eg, renal perfusion) may also occur. The hemodynamic consequences in heart failure patients with reduced EF and in patients with preserved EF can be similar. In patients with preserved EF, the principal mechanism for these hemodynamic changes is increased LV stiffness. By contrast, in patients with reduced EF the principal mechanism is impaired systolic function (**Figure 60**). LV angiography is often unnecessary in patients with heart failure, as noninvasive techniques will have defined the nature and degree of LV dysfunction. However, if performed for clinical reasons, localized hypokinesis (**Figure 61**) or LV dilatation and global hypokinesis in ischemic or nonischemic dilated cardiomyopathy (**Figure 62**) may be seen.

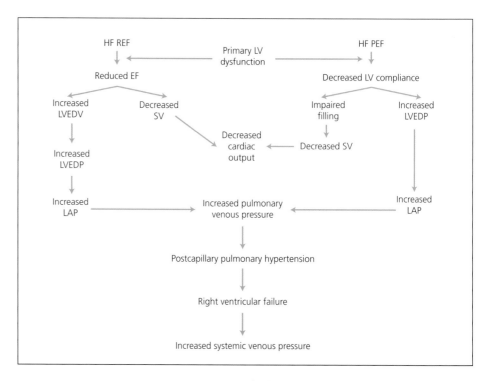

Figure 60. Mechanisms of adverse hemodynamic consequences in heart failure (HF) with reduced ejection fraction (REF) and preserved ejection fraction (PEF). REF results in a reduction in stroke volume (SV) and cardiac output. REF also results in an increase in left ventricular (LV) end-diastolic volume (LVEDV), which is associated with increased LV end-diastolic pressure (LVEDP) and increased left atrial pressure (LAP) and pulmonary venous pressure. The resulting postcapillary pulmonary hypertension may cause right ventricular failure with elevated systemic venous pressure. The hemodynamic consequences in HF PEF are similar to those of HF REF, but the primary initiating factor is decreased LV compliance.

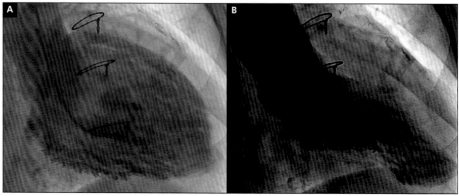

Figure 61. Contrast ventriculogram in right anterior oblique view in a patient with coronary artery disease. End-diastolic (A) and end-systolic (B) frames demonstrate the presence of a left ventricular apical aneurysm.

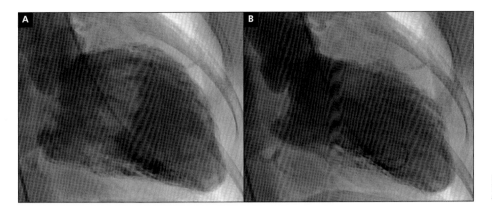

Figure 62. Contrast ventriculogram in right anterior oblique view in a patient with dilated cardiomyopathy. End-diastolic (A) and end-systolic (B) frames demonstrate generalized hypokinesis.

Coronary arteriography is performed to investigate whether heart failure is due to CAD and, if so, to assess the possibilities for treatment (see above). Localized stenoses or, more often, widespread coronary disease may be found (**Figure 63**), even in the absence of a history of an acute coronary syndrome or stable angina. If hibernating myocardium has been demonstrated by nuclear techniques, coronary arteriography is necessary before revascularization can be carried out.

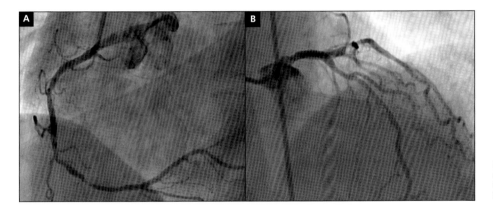

Figure 63. Coronary arteriography in a patient with severe coronary artery disease. There are multiple luminal narrowings of the right coronary artery (A). Left coronary arteriography (B) shows left main and left anterior descending coronary artery stenoses.

Myocardial biopsy

Myocardial biopsy is rarely required to investigate the etiology of heart failure, except to make the diagnosis of giant-cell or fulminant myocarditis, or infiltrative disease such as amyloidosis (**Figure 64**). Currently, the primary indication for myocardial biopsy is to detect rejection following cardiac transplantation.

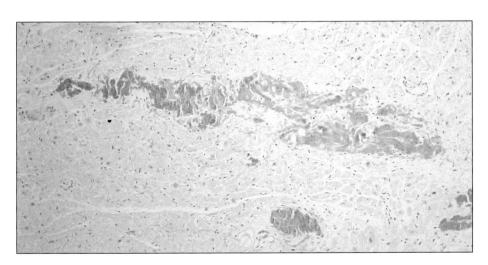

Figure 64. Myocardial biopsy showing amyloid deposition in the myocardium. In congo-red-stained histologic sections, amyloid is a pink homogeneous material. Amyloid is laid down between myocardial cells and ultimately completely surrounds them leaving a lattice of amyloid within which are embedded a few residual muscle cells staining a paler color. Magnification ×150.

Courtesy of M. Sheppard, Royal Brompton Hospital, London.

Epidemiology

ACUTE HEART FAILURE

The European Society of Cardiology has published guidelines for the diagnosis and treatment of acute heart failure [17]. This initiative may result in an increase in epidemiologic information on acute heart failure in the future. However, at the present time epidemiologic information relating to acute heart failure is sparse. Like all epidemiologic information on heart failure, it suffers from the lack of a common, standardized definition of heart failure that allows one study to be compared with another.

It is possible to derive a clinical pattern of patients who have acute heart failure from several surveys carried out both in Europe and in the USA [18–20]. On the basis of these surveys, the typical patient who is admitted with acute heart failure is aged >70 years and equally likely to be male or female.

Approximately half the patients will have a reduced ejection fraction (EF). Acute heart failure patients have many other comorbidities apart from acute heart failure, and many patients presenting with acute heart failure will be admitted to hospital again within 3 months. Hospital stay is longer in Europe than in the USA, and there is a lower rate of re-admission in Europe.

Less than one third of all cases admitted to hospital with acute heart failure are incident cases (*de novo* acute heart failure) [18,20]. In these incident cases, the acute coronary syndrome, usually acute myocardial infarction (MI), is the most frequent etiology. Atrial fibrillation is a common precipitating factor, not only in those cases due to causes other than coronary artery disease (CAD), but even in cases where MI has occurred.

The frequency of heart failure or pulmonary edema, cardiogenic shock, and the risk of hospital death in patients with an acute coronary syndrome has declined significantly. These improvements have been attributed to advances in therapy [21].

EXACERBATIONS OF HEART FAILURE

In the USA, approximately 900,000 patients are admitted to hospital each year because of worsening heart failure [20]. The hospital re-admission rates for patients originally admitted as incident cases of heart failure are high: approximately 20% within 30 days and 50% within 6 months [20]. In Europe, these re-admission rates are due to an exacerbation or worsening of heart failure in approximately 50% of cases [22].

The age and sex distribution, etiology, and precipitating factors for the development of an exacerbation of heart failure requiring hospital admission are the same as for chronic heart failure (see below).

CHRONIC HEART FAILURE

There is significantly more epidemiologic information on chronic heart failure than there is on either acute heart failure or exacerbations of heart failure. However, direct comparisons between different chronic heart failure surveys are also difficult to make because of the inconsistent definition of heart failure used in the various surveys.

PREVALENCE AND INCIDENCE

It has been estimated that approximately 5 million people (2.3%) in the USA have heart failure (*prevalence*) and >550,000 new patients (2 cases per 1,000 of the population) are diagnosed with heart failure each year (*incidence*) [23]. In Europe, the estimates of prevalence range from 0.4% to 2% of the population, and the annual incidence rate is almost 1 case per 1,000 of the population, with a striking rise in rate with increasing age [24].

In developed countries throughout the world, approximately 1–2% of the adult population have heart failure. The incidence and prevalence of heart failure in developing countries is currently unknown, but it might be higher than in developed countries [25].

Information is limited and inconsistent on whether the incidence of heart failure has changed in recent decades. The Framingham Heart Study reported no change for the period 1950–1999 for men, but did show a small fall in the early part of that period for women [26]. Data from Olmsted County, Minnesota, USA showed no change from 1979 to 2000 [27]. The very large Kaiser Permanente database in the Pacific north-west of the USA suggests an increase of 14% in the incidence rate over the two decades from 1970 to 1994 [28]. There are no reliable published data from Europe. It is generally thought that if there is a fall in incidence, the likeliest explanation is the improved treatment of acute MI and hypertension, as both are important causes of heart failure.

AGE AND SEX

In the British population, the median age for incident cases of heart failure is 76 years [19]. The prevalence and incidence of heart failure rises with age (**Figure 65**). The age-adjusted incidence of heart failure is higher in men than in women.

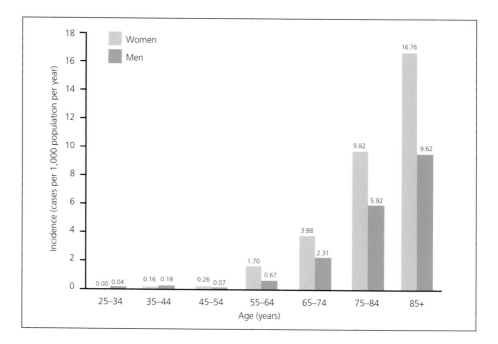

Figure 65. Relationship between the incidence of heart failure and age in a general population. The incidence rises in each decade both in men and women.

Reproduced with permission from the European Society of Cardiology (Cowie MR, Wood DA, Coats AJS, et al. Incidence and aetiology of heart failure. A population-based study. *Eur Heart J* 1999;20:421–8).

ETIOLOGY

There is relatively little information on the etiology of heart failure in unselected populations. The longest established study relating to the epidemiology of heart failure is from Framingham, a small community in Massachusetts, USA. Information on a group of men aged >45 years has been collected over a 60-year period. The group was subsequently enlarged by adding the relatives of the original men who had been included. This study found that hypertension and CAD are the two most common causes of heart failure in the group of patients studied, and that approximately 40% of heart failure cases are due to both causes [29,30].

Registry data suggest that the etiology of acute heart failure and cases of heart failure prevalent in the general population is similar. In the EuroHeart failure survey, CAD followed by valve disease and idiopathic dilated cardiomyopathy were the most common causes of heart failure [18]. Data from the ADHERE (Acute Decompensated Heart Failure National Registry) registry suggest that the cause of heart failure is more likely to be CAD in men than in women (64% vs 51%) [20].

In a survey of a UK population, CAD was found to be the most frequent etiologic factor in incident cases of heart failure [31]. Hypertension, although often co-existing with CAD, was seldom the main reason for the development of heart failure. Such contrasting information between the USA and UK, with respect to hypertension, might reflect the differences between the time periods when the studies were carried out and the use of differing diagnostic techniques for the detection of CAD over these time periods.

Other causes of heart failure in incident cases such as valve disease, congenital heart disease, and cor pulmonale were infrequent in south-east England at the end of the 20th century. One unexpected finding was that a small but significant number of patients had chronic heart failure due to dilated cardiomyopathy, but without CAD.

OBESITY

Obesity is an independent risk factor for the development of heart failure, approximately doubling the risk of heart failure both in men and in women irrespective of the etiology [30,32,33].

THE COST OF HEART FAILURE

The burden of heart failure represents a substantial cost [23]. This has been calculated to consume 1–2% of the total budget of the NHS (National Health Service) in the UK [34]. In the USA, the estimated direct and indirect cost of heart failure in 2006 was $29.6 billion [23].

The largest component of the cost (approximately 60%) is the cost of hospital admissions. These admissions are not only for reasons related to heart failure or its cause, but also for comorbidities in elderly heart failure patients. Other costs include outpatient consultations in hospitals and other clinics, and the cost of treatment. Hospital admissions for heart failure have been increasing in many countries (**Figure 66**) [35], although these admission rates may have reached a plateau in recent years.

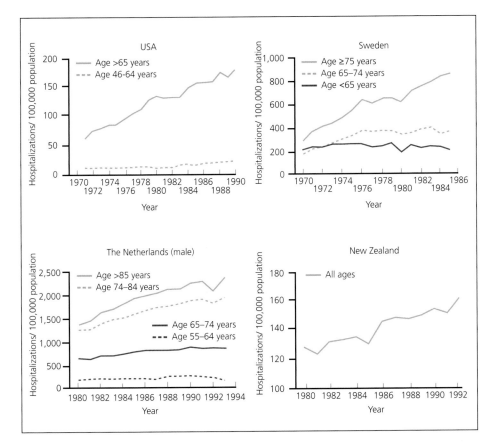

Figure 66. The rise in hospitalizations for heart failure in various countries and in various age groups from year to year.

Reproduced with permission from the European Society of Cardiology (McMurray JJ, Petrie MC, Murdoch DR, et al. Clinical epidemiology of heart failure: public and private health burden. *Eur Heart J* 1998;19(Suppl. P):P9–16).

Management

The objectives of treatment of acute heart failure are to maintain adequate oxygenation, eliminate or decrease pulmonary edema, and improve organ perfusion.

Maintaining adequate oxygenation

Adequate oxygenation is achieved when arterial oxygen saturation becomes normal (95–98%). The airway must be patent, and supplemental oxygen is provided by the administration of increased FiO_2. In the first instance, this is delivered using a face mask or a nasal cannula; if these methods do not correct hypoxia, supplemental oxygen therapy may be delivered through noninvasive ventilation without endotracheal intubation. Either continuous positive airway pressure or noninvasive positive pressure ventilation can be used. Noninvasive ventilation in patients with pulmonary edema improves arterial oxygen saturation, relieves dyspnea, and decreases the need for endotracheal intubation. Mechanical ventilation using endotracheal intubation should be reserved for those patients who do not respond to noninvasive ventilation. It should be appreciated that if the patient is *not* hypoxic, supplemental oxygen therapy can have significant deleterious effects, resulting in decreased coronary blood flow and a reduction in cardiac output.

Eliminating pulmonary edema

In treating acute pulmonary edema, morphine or diamorphine are given to relieve anxiety and the work of breathing. This results in an improvement in breathlessness. Both drugs also decrease the pulmonary capillary wedge pressure. However, they may produce hypotension, and excessive administration can depress the respiratory center.

The intravenous (IV) use of loop diuretics frequently reduces pulmonary congestion and edema, thereby improving breathlessness. The use of diuretics results in natriuresis, increased renal chloride excretion, and secondary enhanced water excretion. Consequently, there is a decrease in intravascular and extracellular volumes. Both pulmonary and systemic venous pressures are reduced.

In acute heart failure, IV loop diuretics can reduce the pulmonary capillary wedge and right atrial pressures within 5–30 minutes due to an increase in venous capacitance, even before diuresis starts. In chronic heart failure (with or without an exacerbation), however, the wedge pressure might actually rise initially due to systemic vasoconstriction from neurohormonal activation.

In patients with pulmonary edema that is resistant to initial therapy (ie, morphine/diamorphine and IV diuretics), continuous infusion of a loop diuretic or combinations of loop diuretics and thiazides may be required. If pulmonary edema persists despite these measures, ultrafiltration might be necessary. Usually such patients also have renal failure.

In all patients with acute heart failure or acute exacerbations of chronic heart failure, irrespective of the etiology, IV nitroglycerine will reduce the pulmonary capillary wedge pressure. Nitroglycerine and nitrates are more effective than diuretics in treating pulmonary edema. They reduce the pulmonary capillary wedge pressure, right atrial pressure, and pulmonary arterial pressure by acting as venodilators. In contrast to diuretics, cardiac output usually remains unchanged. Sublingual or buccal nitroglycerine act very rapidly in this way, and are very useful in the immediate treatment of pulmonary venous congestion. However, the development of tolerance is a significant problem with the use both of nitroglycerine and of other nitrates.

Sodium nitroprusside acts similarly to nitroglycerine in reducing the pulmonary capillary wedge, right atrial, and pulmonary arterial pressures. In contrast to nitroglycerine, however, it also *increases* cardiac output by reducing systemic vascular resistance. This is because sodium nitroprusside is a balanced arterial and venodilator, whereas nitroglycerine is predominantly a venodilator. Consequently, nitroprusside is particularly useful in patients who have a reduced cardiac output and increased systemic vascular resistance. If, in addition, such a patient has mitral regurgitation, the degree of regurgitation will be reduced by the reduction in systemic vascular resistance.

Improving organ perfusion

Positive inotropic agents such as dobutamine (a β_1 agonist), milrinone and enoximone (inodilators), or levosimendan (a calcium-sensitizing agent) are sometimes used in acute heart failure to improve cardiac output and organ perfusion. All positive inotropic agents potentially increase the risk of arrhythmias and mortality. In patients who are significantly hypotensive, vasopressor agents such as dopamine, norepinephrine, or phenylephrine can be used in addition to the positive inotropic agents.

Cardiac glycosides such as digitalis exert their positive inotropic action by inhibiting myocardial sodium/potassium ATPase. They are weakly positive inotropic agents and are seldom used in the treatment of acute heart failure. Like most other positive inotropic agents they increase myocardial oxygen consumption. However, digitalis has a place in the treatment of patients with atrial fibrillation precipitating acute heart failure.

Management of arrhythmias

Patients who present with acute heart failure frequently do so because of the development of arrhythmias. Prompt treatment of the arrhythmia is important. Direct current (DC) cardioversion may be required to convert atrial fibrillation to sinus rhythm following anticoagulation. In patients with a reduced ejection fraction (EF), amiodarone is the most effective agent for maintaining sinus rhythm. Amiodarone is also the most effective agent for treating atrial flutter or supraventricular tachycardia if DC cardioversion is not to be used. Catheter-based ablation after stabilization is the most effective way of preventing recurrence. Digitalis, with or without additional β-blockers or amiodarone, in order to control the ventricular rate in patients who remain in atrial fibrillation.

Ventricular arrhythmias usually require immediate DC cardioversion. Amiodarone is the drug of choice for the prevention of recurrence. An implantable cardioverter-defibrillator (ICD) is frequently placed after the patient has stabilized.

The usual treatment of symptomatic bradyarrhythmias is the immediate insertion of a temporary pacemaker, although atropine is sometimes effective. Permanent pacemaker insertion should normally be considered after the patient has stabilized.

Anticoagulation, initially with heparin and subsequently with oral anticoagulants, is indicated in patients who have atrial fibrillation or flutter. There is controversy over the use of anticoagulants in patients who have heart failure with a reduced EF and who are in sinus rhythm. However, those who have systemic or pulmonary embolism require anticoagulation.

Acute heart failure complicating acute coronary syndromes

Approximately 25% of patients with acute coronary syndromes (acute MI and unstable angina) develop heart failure. The mortality of these patients is high. Heart failure or cardiogenic shock occur most frequently in patients with ST-segment elevation MI (STEMI), but also occur in a small proportion of those with unstable angina or non-ST-segment MI (NSTEMI). The mortality of patients who develop cardiogenic shock is approximately 55%, despite the use of a variety of aggressive treatments.

In patients with STEMI, percutaneous coronary intervention (PCI) should be considered. In those who are not suitable for such a procedure, coronary artery bypass surgery and intra-aortic balloon counterpulsation (IABP) should be considered. If PCI is not immediately available, fibrinolytic therapy should be applied and the patient transferred to a center where more specialized invasive treatment is available. PCI should also be considered in patients with heart failure due to unstable angina or NSTEMI.

Patients with heart failure complicating acute coronary syndromes who are considered for PCI are normally treated with aspirin and clopidogrel, and sometimes with additional glycoprotein IIb/IIIa antagonists. Low-molecular-weight or unfractionated heparin is used as an antithrombotic agent.

Angiotensin-converting enzyme (ACE) inhibitors or angiotensin II receptor blockers (ARBs) have been shown to affect favorably the prognosis of patients with acute MI. This is particularly true of patients whose MI is complicated by the development of heart failure. However, ACE inhibitors are contraindicated in patients with cardiogenic shock. ACE inhibitors should be continued indefinitely in patients with a reduced EF following an MI.

β-blockers should be given to all patients following an MI, irrespective of whether the infarct was complicated by heart failure. However, they are contraindicated in patients with cardiogenic shock, hypotension, or bradycardia, or if the patient is likely to develop bronchospasm.

Some patients with an acute MI develop heart failure as a result of mechanical complications. These include rupture or dysfunction of the papillary muscles, which results in severe mitral regurgitation, or rupture of the ventricular septum. These patients usually develop severe heart failure, and have a particularly high mortality rate. Surgical intervention is usually required following a time period during which the patient is supported by IABP or possibly by using sodium nitroprusside. Repair or replacement of the mitral valve is the definitive treatment for mitral regurgitation. The ruptured septum may be closed by either surgery or via a catheter technique. The general principles of the treatment of acute heart failure are summarized in **Table 6**.

Table 6. Summary of management of acute heart failure.
Maintain adequate oxygenation
Eliminate pulmonary edema
– Morphine/diamorphine
– Diuretics
– Nitrates/sodium nitroprusside
Improve organ perfusion
– Positive inotropic agents
Management of arrhythmias
Management of acute coronary syndromes

CHRONIC HEART FAILURE

The management of patients who have chronic heart failure due to valvular or congenital heart disease involves consideration of surgery, while those who have cor pulmonale require treatment of the underlying cause. The following sections apply to patients who have chronic heart failure due to myocardial disease with a *reduced EF*.

Specialized support services

The development of specialized services for patients with different cardiologic problems has occurred over a long period of time, following the introduction of pacemaker clinics in the 1960s. Such services for patients with heart failure now include specialized clinics, both in hospitals and in primary care, that are usually run by highly trained nurses with the support of doctors who are experienced in dealing with chronic heart failure patients. Patients who live at home have telephone access to specialized nurses who can provide immediate advice on care or make appropriate referrals to other services. These services also provide advice on the adjustment of diuretic doses, adherence to recommended treatment, diet, and physical activity. Advice is also provided on the need to either call emergency services or attend outpatient clinics for evaluation.

The value of these support services has been assessed. Comparisons have been made between conventional outpatient care in general clinics and care in specialized heart failure clinics. These comparisons have shown a better outcome for patients who receive care in the specialized clinics. Management by these services has been shown to reduce the rate of hospitalization and to improve quality of life and survival [36].

Risk factor management

Patients who have risk factors for the development of heart failure, or for the premature development of CAD (which may lead to heart failure), should have appropriate treatment of such risk factors. Thus, weight reduction is important in obese patients because obesity is a risk factor for the development of heart failure. Similarly, cessation of smoking and control of diabetes, hypertension, and hyperlipidemia should be part of the management of patients with CAD. The importance of statins in reducing mortality in patients with CAD has been established by landmark trials [37]. Recent trials have shown that statin therapy reduces mortality in chronic heart failure with a reduced EF, irrespective of whether it is due to CAD or other causes [38].

Pharmacologic treatment

The treatment of chronic heart failure aims to control symptoms (breathlessness and fatigue), to control fluid retention and prevent fluid accumulation, and to improve prognosis. A wide variety of pharmacologic agents may be used in patients with chronic heart failure. These include diuretics, vasodilators, ACE inhibitors, β-blockers, ARBs, positive inotropic agents, aldosterone inhibitors, calcium-channel blockers, antiarrhythmic agents, and anticoagulants. Each of these pharmacologic agents will be considered with respect to the objectives of treatment.

Diuretics

Fluid retention is most likely to be relieved with diuretics. For maintenance therapy, oral loop diuretics are used (furosemide [frusemide], bumetanide, or torasemide [torsemide]), as well as thiazides or potassium-sparing diuretics (aldosterone antagonists or amiloride). In very severe fluid retention that is unresponsive to either oral or IV furosemide, a combination of loop diuretics, thiazides, and aldosterone antagonists may be used. The prevention of fluid reaccumulation, once it has been relieved, is critically dependent on the continued use of diuretics; however, the appropriate maintenance dose is difficult to establish. A dose of diuretics that is too high will produce hypovolemia (which may result in dizziness or syncope due to hypotension) and renal failure, while a dose that is too low can lead to the reaccumulation of fluid.

The symptoms of breathlessness and fatigue are unaffected by diuretics in patients with chronic heart failure but without pulmonary edema. Increasing the dose of diuretics in patients who have neither peripheral nor pulmonary edema in an attempt to improve breathlessness will result in hypovolemia and worsening renal failure. Furthermore, diuretic therapy may adversely stimulate the neurohormonal systems.

There is no evidence that diuretic treatment affects the prognosis or survival rate of patients with chronic heart failure.

Vasodilators

Although vasodilators such as nitroglycerine and other nitrates reduce acute pulmonary congestion by virtue of reducing the pulmonary capillary wedge and right atrial pressures, there is no good evidence from clinical trials that they improve symptoms in patients with chronic heart failure.

Nitric oxide-enhancing agents (a combination of the direct-acting vasodilators hydralazine and isosorbide dinitrate) were originally shown to improve mortality rates in patients with chronic heart failure [39], but not as effectively as ACE inhibitors (see next section) [40]. However, more recently, a large clinical trial in black patients demonstrated that the addition of hydralazine and isosorbide dinitrate to the standard pharmacologic treatment of chronic heart failure due to myocardial dysfunction with reduced EF is associated with significant reductions in death from any cause and the number of patients hospitalized for heart failure. There was also an improvement in quality of life (**Figure 67**) [41].

Endpoint	Isosorbide dinitrate plus hydralazine (n=518)	Placebo (n=532)	P value
Primary composite score[a]	−0.1±1.9	−0.5±2.0	0.01
Components of the primary composite score			
Death from any cause — n (%)	32 (6.2)	54 (10.2)	0.02
First hospitalization for heart failure — n (%)	85 (16.4)	130 (24.4)	0.001
Change in quality-of-life score at 6 months[b]	−5.6±20.6	−2.7±21.2	0.02

Figure 67. Primary composite score results of a randomized trial comparing isosorbide dinitrate plus hydralazine treatment versus placebo in black patients with advanced heart failure. Plus-minus values are means±standard deviations. [a]Scores can range from −6 to 2, with higher scores indicating a better outcome. [b]Lower scores indicate a better quality of life.

Reproduced with permission from Massachusetts Medical Society (Taylor AL, Ziesche RN, Yancy C, et al. Combination of isosorbide dinitrate and hydralazine in blacks with heart failure. N Engl J Med 2004;351:2049–57).

ACE inhibitors

Many clinical trials have demonstrated the value of ACE inhibitors in patients with chronic heart failure. Although a meta-analysis of placebo-controlled ACE inhibitor trials has suggested that breathlessness is improved with ACE inhibitor therapy [42], the main role of this therapy lies in improving prognosis and mortality rates (**Figure 68**).

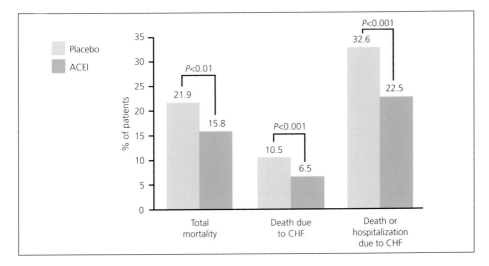

Figure 68. Results of a pooled analysis of 32 randomized trials of treatment with angiotensin-converting enzyme inhibitors (ACEIs) in heart failure with reduced ejection fraction. Compared with placebo, treatment with ACEIs was associated with a significant reduction in total mortality, death due to congestive heart failure (CHF) and in the death or hospitalization due to CHF.

The importance of ACE inhibitors in patients with severe chronic heart failure was established by the landmark CONSENSUS (Cooperative North Scandinavian Enalapril Survival Study) trial [43]. Subsequently, these observations were confirmed by several other trials. The improvement in prognosis with ACE inhibitors was also demonstrated in symptomatic patients in the SOLVD (Studies of Left Ventricular Dysfunction) trial. However, no prognostic benefit was found in asymptomatic patients with LV dysfunction (mainly due to previous MI) [44]. Patients with asymptomatic LV systolic dysfunction following MI had a reduced risk for developing heart failure and reduced mortality when treated with an ACE inhibitor (**Figure 69**) [45].

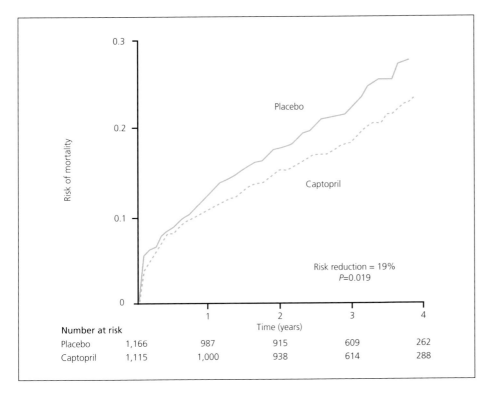

Figure 69. Effect of treatment with captopril on mortality rate in patients with left ventricular systolic dysfunction following acute myocardial infarction.

Reproduced with permission from Massachusetts Medical Society (Pfeffer MA, Braunwald E, Moy LA, et al. Effect of captopril on mortality and morbidity in patients with left-ventricular dysfunction after myocardial infarction: results of the survival and ventricular enlargement trial. *N Engl J Med* 1992;327:669–77).

The use of ACE inhibitors may be restricted by unwanted effects. Hypotension can occur, so initial exposure to these agent needs to be handled cautiously. Patients who are hypovolemic are at particular risk because of hypotension. Hyperkalemia and worsening renal function can also occur; potassium blood levels and renal function should be monitored, and the concomitant use of potassium-sparing diuretics or potassium supplements avoided. A history of peripheral vascular disease should alert the clinician to the possibility that the patient has additional renal vascular disease; in this situation, renal failure can be precipitated by the introduction of ACE inhibitors.

Cough and loss of taste can limit the use of ACE inhibitors. Hypersensitivity reactions, such as the development of angioedema, may be life-threatening. ACE inhibitors are contraindicated in pregnancy because of the possible development of fetal abnormalities.

β-Blockers

Clinical trials have shown that β-blockers have a beneficial effect on prognosis in patients with chronic heart failure and reduced EF. Reductions in mortality have been demonstrated with various β-blockers, and the overall benefit has been demonstrated in a meta-analysis (**Figure 70**) [46]. This improvement in mortality has even been observed in the most severely symptomatic patients [47]. Long-term β-blocker therapy, when tolerated, has been shown to be associated with an improvement in functional class and quality of life [48].

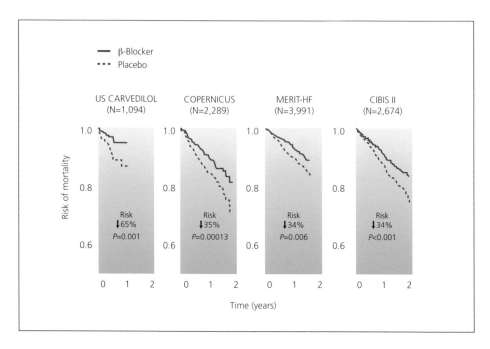

Figure 70. Effects of β-blocker therapy in patients with heart failure and reduced ejection fraction in four randomized clinical trials. Compared with placebo, treatment with carvedilol, a nonselective β-blocker with α-adrenergic blocking and antioxidant properties, decreased the risk of mortality both in the US CARVEDILOL and COPERNICUS trials. In the CIBIS II trial, bisoprolol, a selective β-blocker with vasodilating properties, and in the MERIT-HF trial, metoprolol CR/XL, a selective slow release and long acting β-blocker, have also been shown to decrease mortality.

β-blocker therapy reduces the risk of sudden cardiac death [47–49]. β-blockers can also have a beneficial effect in reducing exercise-induced rises in heart rate and causing a consequent improvement in ventricular filling. In a comparative study, a nonselective β-blocker with α-adrenergic-blocking properties (carvedilol) has been shown to improve survival to a significantly greater degree than a selective, short-acting, immediate-release β-blocker (metoprolol) [50].

Angiotensin II receptor blockers

The initial clinical trials of ARBs were mainly carried out to compare the effects of these agents with ACE inhibitors. Mortality rates were not significantly different between these agents [51,52]. In a noncomparative, randomly allocated, placebo-controlled trial, the ARB candesartan was shown to reduce mortality and morbidity (including hospital admissions) in patients with chronic heart failure (**Figure 71**) [53]. ARBs have also been shown to improve quality of life [52].

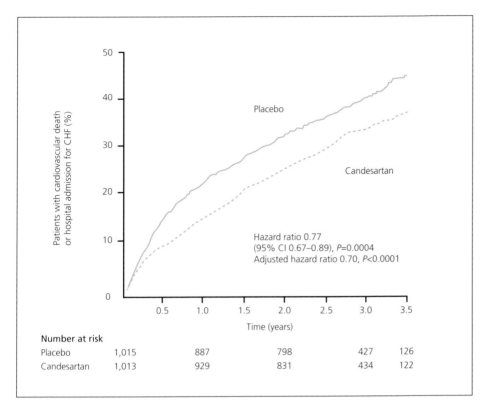

Figure 71. Effect of treatment with the angiotensin receptor-blocking agent candesartan on cardiovascular death or hospital admission in patients with congestive heart failure (CHF) and reduced ejection fraction.

Reproduced with permission from Elsevier, Inc. (Granger CB, McMurray JJ, Yusuf S, et al. for the CHARM Investigators and Committees. Effects of candesartan in patients with chronic heart failure and reduced left-ventricular systolic function intolerant to angiotensin-converting-enzyme inhibitors: the CHARM-Alternative trial. *Lancet* 2003;362:772–6).

Because ARBs rarely have the same unwanted effects as ACE inhibitors (cough and angioedema), it is appropriate to use them in patients who have side effects with ACE inhibitors.

The addition of an ARB (candesartan) to ACE inhibitor therapy has been associated with a reduction in hospital admissions [54]. However, such combination therapy may increase the risk of hypotension and worsening renal failure.

Positive inotropic agents: digitalis
The use of digitalis preparations to control the heart rate in chronic heart failure patients who are in atrial fibrillation is not controversial. However, there is controversy regarding the value of digitalis in chronic heart failure patients who are in sinus rhythm. In a placebo-controlled trial, in which digoxin was added to conventional medical therapy, digoxin taken in an oral dose resulting in a blood level of ≤1.1 ng/mL was shown to improve symptoms and frequency of hospital admissions, but did not reduce mortality rates [55]. However, arrhythmogenic activity was increased in patients with a digoxin blood level of >1.1 ng/mL.

Other positive inotropic agents
There is a place for the short-term use of other positive inotropic agents (eg, dobutamine, dopamine, milrinone, enoximone) in an attempt to produce clinical improvement in the extremely ill patient, usually with worsening or decompensated heart failure. However, the evidence from clinical trials suggests that these agents, if

continued for a prolonged period, may carry an adverse effect on survival rates in patients with chronic heart failure [56].

Aldosterone inhibitors

The aldosterone inhibitor spironolactone has been shown to be a useful agent in patients with severe chronic heart failure. A large, placebo-controlled study (the RALES [Randomized Aldactone Evaluation Study] trial) has shown that spironolactone has a beneficial effect on overall survival and risk of sudden cardiac death in patients with chronic heart failure (**Figure 72**) [57].

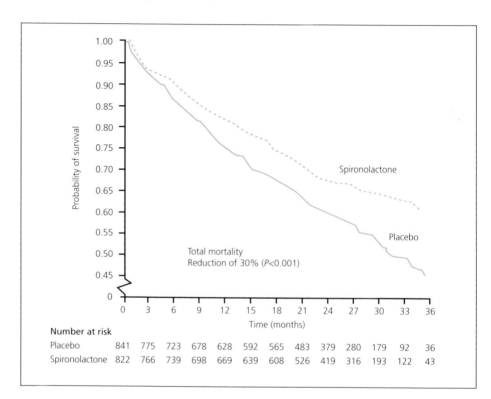

Figure 72. Comparison of the aldosterone antagonist spironolactone and placebo in patients with heart failure and reduced ejection fraction (RALES trial).

Reproduced with permission from Massachusetts Medical Society (Pitt B, Zannad F, Remme W, et al. The effect of spironolactone on mortality and morbidity in patients with severe heart failure. *N Engl J Med* 1999;341:709–17).

Calcium-channel blockers

There is no evidence that calcium-channel blockers, which act predominantly as vasodilators, improve survival in patients with chronic heart failure [58]. There is also no evidence that calcium-channel blockers, which control the heart rate and theoretically increase diastolic filling, have any beneficial effect.

Antiarrhythmic agents

Approximately 30% of patients with chronic heart failure and reduced EF have atrial fibrillation. The prevalence of atrial flutter or other supraventricular tachycardias is much lower. Amiodarone is the drug of choice to maintain sinus rhythm in patients with paroxysmal atrial tachyarrhythmias. Class IC drugs are contraindicated. Class III drugs such as sotalol (which has additional β-blocker properties) and dofetilide are sometimes used, but these carry a risk of polymorphous ventricular tachycardia.

Catheter-based ablation therapy has been shown to improve EF in some patients with permanent atrial fibrillation. In patients with atrial fibrillation and an uncontrolled ventricular rate despite the use of appropriate drugs, atrioventricular junctional ablation and a permanent pacemaker are occasionally required.

In patients with paroxysmal ventricular tachycardia, an ICD is required (see below), but amiodarone might also be required to decrease the frequency of ICD discharge.

Anticoagulants

In patients who have chronic heart failure with atrial fibrillation, the risk of systemic embolism is reduced by maintenance anticoagulant treatment [59]. Patients who are in sinus rhythm may benefit from maintenance anticoagulant treatment. However, there is no certain evidence that they do, while the risk of bleeding is undoubtedly raised. Aspirin therapy, which is frequently used in those patients with CAD, is not necessarily helpful in those with chronic heart failure who are on other pharmacologic agents such as ACE inhibitors.

The pharmacologic treatment of patients with chronic heart failure and reduced EF is summarized in **Table 7**.

Table 7. Pharmacologic treatment of chronic heart failure with reduced ejection fraction.
Diuretics
Vasodilators
Angiotensin-converting enzyme inhibitors
β-blockers
Angiotensin II receptor blockers
Digitalis and other positive inotropic agents
Aldosterone inhibitors
Calcium-channel blockers
Antiarrhythmic agents
Anticoagulants

ADVANCED HEART FAILURE

Advanced heart failure describes the condition of patients who continue to experience severe symptoms, often requiring repetitive hospital admissions despite pharmacologic therapy. A variety of treatments, using both conventional surgery and device therapy, have been developed in an attempt to improve the quality of life of these patients and reduce mortality.

Conventional surgical treatment

A variety of surgical procedures have been attempted in patients with chronic heart failure. The patient who remains significantly symptomatic despite medical treatment and who has a localized left ventricular (LV) aneurysm following an earlier acute MI may benefit from aneurysmectomy, with or without revascularization. Mitral valve repair in selected patients and LV constraining devices are currently undergoing clinical trials. Partial left ventriculectomy, with or without mitral valve repair, in patients with a dilated cardiomyopathy that is not due to CAD (the Baptista procedure) has largely been abandoned.

In patients whose heart failure is due to a dilated cardiomyopathy as a result of CAD, EF has been shown to improve with revascularization [60]. However, revascularization, either by PCI or by coronary artery bypass surgery, will only improve the mechanical function of the left ventricle if hibernating (viable) myocardium is present. The presence of hibernating myocardium can be established using thallium myocardial perfusion imaging or dipyridamole sestamibi nuclear scanning, positron emission tomography, magnetic resonance imaging (MRI), or dobutamine stress echocardiography.

Although there is a theoretical advantage in revascularizing hibernating myocardium in patients with severe heart failure, a randomized clinical trial has yet to be performed in this patient group.

Device treatment

Device treatment for patients with chronic heart failure due to myocardial dysfunction includes cardiac resynchronization therapy (CRT), ICD, an LV assist device, and enhanced external counterpulsation (EECP).

Cardiac resynchronization therapy

CRT involves the use of atrial-synchronized biventricular pacing. Approximately a third of patients with chronic heart failure due to myocardial dysfunction have an electrocardiographic QRS duration of >120 ms, usually seen as left bundle branch block. In such patients, ventricular dyssynchrony is present resulting in further LV dysfunction. In patients with severe chronic heart failure due to systolic dysfunction and reduced EF, CRT has been shown to reduce hospital admissions and increase the duration of survival compared with conventional treatment without CRT (CARE-HF [Cardiac Resynchronization-Heart Failure] trial) (**Figure 73**) [61].

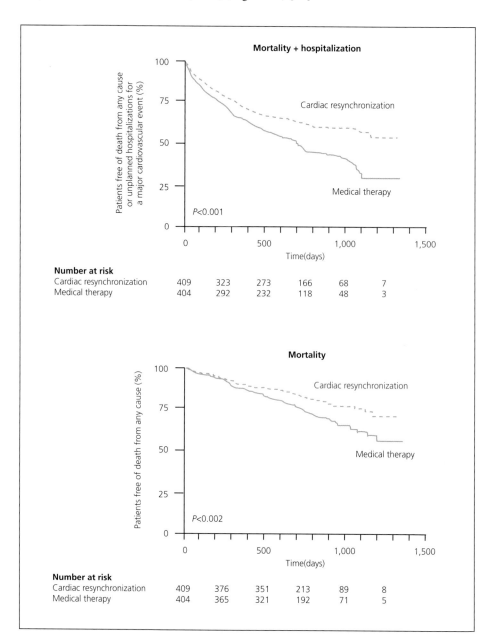

Figure 73. Effect of cardiac resynchronization treatment compared with medical treatment alone in patients with heart failure and reduced ejection fraction (CARE-HF trial).

Reproduced with permission from Massachusetts Medical Society (Cleland JG, Daubert JC, Erdmann E, et al. Cardiac Resynchronization – Heart Failure (CARE-HF) Study Investigators. The effect of cardiac resynchronization on morbidity and mortality in heart failure. *N Engl J Med* 2005;352:1539–49).

Even patients with a normal QRS duration can have mechanical dyssynchrony, and some of these patients might also benefit from CRT. In patients with severe chronic heart failure with reduced EF, CRT with an ICD has been shown to significantly reduce rates of mortality and hospitalization for heart failure compared with optimal medical treatment (**Figure 74**) [62]. However, patients with chronic heart failure and preserved EF have *not* been shown to benefit from CRT.

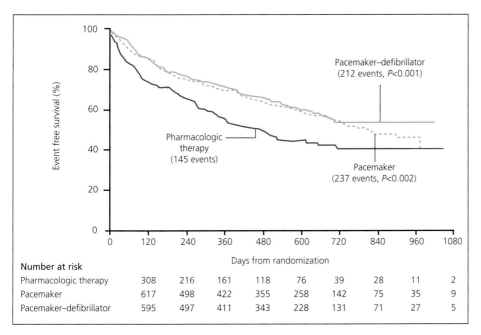

Figure 74. Results of cardiac resynchronization alone and cardiac resynchronization and implantable cardioverter-defibrillator compared with pharmacologic therapy in patients with severe heart failure and reduced ejection fraction (COMPANION trial).

Reproduced with permission from Massachusetts Medical Society (Bristow MR, Saxon LA, Boehmer J, et al. Cardiac resynchronization therapy with or without an implantable defibrillator in advanced chronic heart failure. *N Engl J Med* 2004;350:2140–50).

The most frequent technique used to determine whether mechanical dyssynchrony is present is tissue Doppler imaging. Alternatively, cardiac MRI can also be used. It is crucial to determine whether mechanical dyssynchrony is present in order to select patients who may benefit from CRT.

Implantable cardioverter-defibrillator

Patients with chronic heart failure often die suddenly, probably due to the development of ventricular fibrillation. For that reason, ICD devices are used as part of the management of seriously ill heart failure patients. A comparative trial involving single-lead ICD versus amiodarone and placebo demonstrated a benefit for those patients randomly allocated to the ICD device, with a significant reduction in mortality rate in comparison with either amiodarone or placebo (**Figure 75**) [63]. The mortality rates with amiodarone and placebo were the same. The trial involved patients with moderately severe heart failure of both ischemic and nonischemic etiologies and reduced EF.

In patients with reduced EF following an MI, those randomly assigned to an ICD had a lower mortality rate than those managed with conventional medical therapy alone [64].

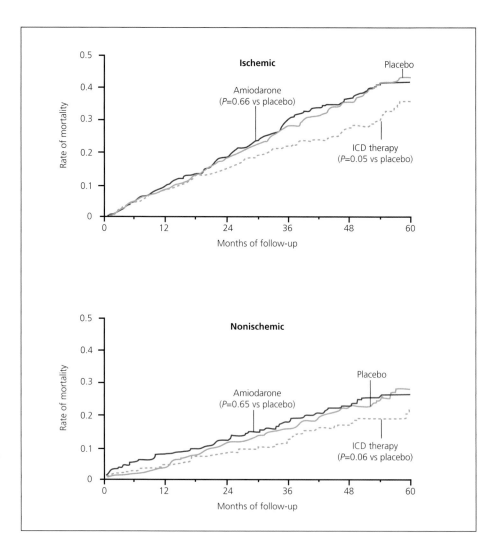

Figure 75. Effect of implantable cardioverter-defibrillator (ICD) therapy compared with placebo or amiodarone on the mortality rate of patients with heart failure and reduced ejection fraction. In patients with ischemic (top) and nonischemic (bottom) cardiomyopathy, ICD therapy was associated with a lower mortality rate (SCD-HeFT trial).

Reproduced with permission from Massachusetts Medical Society (Brady GH, Lee KL, Mark DB, et al. Amiodarone or an implantable cardioverter-defibrillator for congestive heart failure. *N Engl J Med* 2005;352:225–37).

Left ventricular assist devices

Implantable LV assist devices or mechanical support systems have been used for some time to support the patient with advanced heart failure until cardiac transplantation can be carried out. The shortage of donors prompted trials in patients who were ineligible for cardiac transplantation. One such trial showed that patients with advanced heart failure who were randomly allocated to an LV assist device had a significantly higher rate of survival than those allocated to medical therapy alone. The frequency of serious adverse events (infection, bleeding, and malfunction of the device) was higher than in the medical therapy group [65].

Enhanced external counterpulsation

EECP involves the sequential inflation and deflation of three sets of lower extremity cuffs. As in IABP, there is augmentation of diastolic blood pressure. This increases coronary blood flow and reduces the impedance to systole, which increases cardiac output. It also increases venous return. In a multicenter randomized trial, patients with chronic heart failure and reduced EF demonstrated increased exercise capacity, exercise duration, functional class, and peak oxygen consumption with this therapy. However, there was no benefit with respect to survival [66].

Cardiac transplantation

Cardiac transplantation for suitable patients with advanced heart failure is carried out in many international centers, and is associated with satisfactory survival rates: the 1-year, 5-year, and 10-year survival rates are approximately 80%, 70%, and 50%, respectively (**Figure 76**) [67]. Over the years, the improvement in survival rates has been mainly due to improvements in immunosuppressive therapy. However, cardiac transplantation is severely limited by the shortage of donors. It is estimated that approximately 3,000 cardiac transplants are carried out worldwide each year. The nonpharmacologic treatment of advanced heart failure with reduced EF is summarized in **Table 8**.

Table 8. Nonpharmacologic treatment of advanced heart failure with reduced ejection fraction.
Conventional surgical treatment
Left ventricular aneurysmectomy
Mitral valve repair
Revascularization of hibernating myocardium
Partial left ventriculectomy
Cardiac resynchronization therapy
Implantable cardioverter-defibrillator
Left ventricular assist devices
Enhanced external counterpulsation
Cardiac transplantation

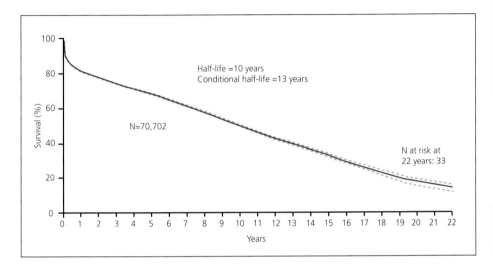

Figure 76. International survival for heart transplantation (1984–2005). Reproduced with permission from Elsevier, Inc. (Taylor DO, Edwards LB, Boucek MM, et al. Registry of the International Society for Heart and Lung Transplantation: twenty-fourth official adult heart transplantation report – 2007. *J Heart Lung Transplant* 2007;26:769–81.

CHRONIC HEART FAILURE WITH PRESERVED EJECTION FRACTION

Clinical trials have not demonstrated an improved prognosis with the use of pharmacologic agents in patients with chronic heart failure and preserved EF. However, hospital re-admission rates may be reduced by the use of ARBs [68]. In addition, symptoms can be improved with drugs that slow the ventricular rate. A rapid heart rate is associated with impaired ventricular filling and consequent hemodynamic deterioration; thus, slowing the heart rate with β-blockers, amiodarone, or heart-rate regulating calcium-channel blockers can be symptomatically beneficial. The maintenance of sinus rhythm is important. Paroxysmal atrial fibrillation can be prevented with amiodarone. Patients who have atrial fibrillation with an uncontrolled ventricular rate can be treated with digoxin, β-blockers, or calcium-channel blockers, with or without additional amiodarone. If such pharmacologic treatment is unsuccessful the patient may be considered for atrioventricular junctional ablation together with right ventricular permanent pacing in an attempt to improve his/her symptoms.

In hypertensive patients, control of hypertension can improve ventricular relaxation and, consequently, symptoms. Aldosterone antagonists may decrease myocardial fibrosis. In patients with overt myocardial ischemia, drugs that relieve myocardial ischemia can be useful. Fluid retention requires the use of diuretics and, possibly, aldosterone antagonists.

The role of CRT in patients with chronic heart failure and preserved EF who have mechanical dyssynchrony has not been established. The management of patients with chronic heart failure with preserved EF is summarized in **Table 9**.

Table 9. Management of chronic heart failure with preserved ejection fraction
Maintain sinus rhythm (amiodarone)
Control ventricular rate in atrial fibrillation (digitalis, β-blockers, calcium-channel blockers, amiodarone)
Atrioventricular junctional ablation and right ventricular permanent pacing if ventricular rate is uncontrolled in atrial fibrillation
Control hypertension
Control fluid retention (diuretics, aldosterone antagonists)
Control myocardial ischemia
Reduce hospital admissions (angiotensin II receptor blockers)

Prognosis

The prevalence of individuals who have systolic dysfunction with reduced ejection fraction (EF) in the community has been determined in Olmsted County, Minnesota, USA by carrying out echocardiographic screening studies [69]. The estimated prevalence was between 2% and 6%. By contrast, a population screening study in Glasgow, UK revealed that 1.4% of a population of 1,467 individuals aged 25–74 years had asymptomatic left ventricular systolic dysfunction [70]. The prognosis in such individuals is not benign: the percentage of individuals with a diagnosis of overt heart failure ranges from 20% to 45% [69], and the average annual mortality rate lies between 5% and 10%.

PATIENTS WITH HEART FAILURE, LEFT VENTRICULAR DYSFUNCTION, AND REDUCED EJECTION FRACTION

The prognosis in patients with heart failure, left ventricular dysfunction, and reduced EF has been shown to be associated with a number of factors [71]. A worse prognosis is associated with male gender, increasing age, increasing severity of symptoms, acute coronary syndromes as the etiology, systemic hypotension, impaired renal function, hyponatremia, and raised B-type natriuretic peptide levels. Comorbidities, especially diabetes mellitus, anemia, and pulmonary disease, also affect prognosis adversely (**Table 10**).

In spite of the wide range of therapies for heart failure described in **Management**, mortality rates remain high. The mortality rates for patients with heart failure are often compared to those for cancer; the mortality rate in England is similar to that of bowel cancer, and worse than for breast cancer [72]. In unselected European populations of cases of incident heart failure, the survival rates are approximately 63%, 51%, and 35% at 1, 2, and 5 years, respectively (**Figure 77**) [73]. Similar rates are reported from the USA [26]. Mortality is particularly high in the first month following presentation.

There is evidence that mortality rates in patients with reduced EFs have fallen in recent years both in the USA [26,74] and in the UK [75]. This may be attributed to the use of modern pharmacologic agents, particularly angiotensin-converting enzyme inhibitors and β-blockers, or improvement in the treatment of acute coronary syndromes.

Table 10. Adverse prognostic features.

Adverse prognostic features
Male gender
Increasing age
Increasing severity of symptoms
Acute coronary syndromes causing heart failure
Systemic hypotension
Impaired renal function
Hyponatremia
Raised B-type natriuretic peptide
Comorbidities, especially diabetes mellitus, anemia, and pulmonary disease

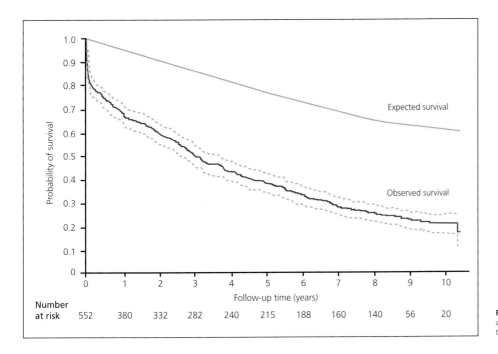

Figure 77. The observed survival of incident cases of heart failure in a general population (London heart failure cohort) compared with the expected survival of individuals in a similar age group.

The main modes of death in patients with chronic heart failure are sudden death and progressive heart failure [76]. Death from noncardiovascular causes is also common in these patients. All these mortality rates increase with decreasing EF (**Figure 78**) [77].

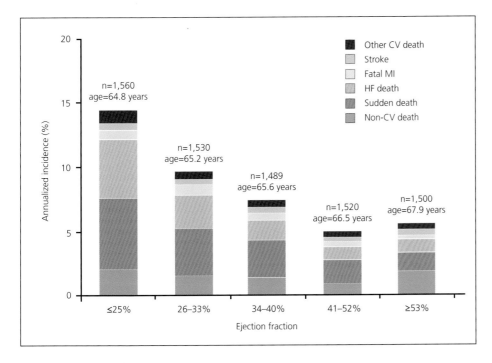

Figure 78. The annualized incidence of mortality in patients with heart failure in relation to ejection fraction. CV: cardiovascular; HF: heart failure; MI: myocardial infarction; Non-CV: noncardiovascular.

Reproduced with permission from the American College of Cardiology (Solomon S, Olofsson B, Finn P, et al. Cause of death across full spectrum of ventricular function in patients with heart failure: the CHARM study. *J Am Coll Cardiol* 2004,43[Suppl. 1]:180 [abstr.]).

PATIENTS WITH HEART FAILURE, LEFT VENTRICULAR DYSFUNCTION, AND PRESERVED EJECTION FRACTION

There is inadequate information available to comment on this group of patients [10]. However, there are serial community echo-Doppler studies that suggest an unfavorable prognosis. In these studies, mild diastolic dyfunction was associated with an 8-fold increase in the risk of death and severe dysfunction with a 10-fold increase [69]. In selected patients with chronic heart failure the annual mortality rate is approximately 4% in mild to moderate heart failure and rises with more severe heart failure [68]. Unlike patients with a reduced EF, advances in therapy do not appear to have made any improvement in the prognosis of patients with preserved EF [78].

References

1. Lewis T. *Diseases of the Heart*. London: MacMillan,1933.
2. Task Force on Heart Failure of the European Society of Cardiology: Guidelines for the diagnosis of heart failure. *Eur Heart J* 1995;16:741–51.
3. Braunwald E. Heart Disease. In: *Textbook of Cardiovascular Medicine*. Philadelphia: WB Saunders, 1980.
4. Poole-Wilson PA. Heart Failure. *Med Intern* 1985;2:866–71.
5. Swedberg K, Cleland J, Dargie H, et al. Guidelines for the diagnosis and treatment of chronic heart failure: executive summary (update 2005): The Task Force for the Diagnosis and Treatment of Chronic Heart Failure of the European Society of Cardiology. *Eur Heart J* 2005;26:1115–40.
6. Aurigemma GP, Zile MR, Gaasch WH. Contractile behavior of the left ventricle in diastolic heart failure: with emphasis on regional systolic function. *Circulation* 2006;113:296–304.
7. van Heerebeek L, Borbely A, Niessen HW, et al. Myocardial structure and function differ in systolic and diastolic heart failure. *Circulation* 2006;113:1966–73.
8. Katz AM, Zile MR. New molecular mechanism in diastolic heart failure. *Circulation* 2006;113:1922–5.
9. Zile MR, Baicu CF, Gaasch WH. Diastolic heart failure-abnormalities in active relaxation and passive stiffness of the left ventricle. *N Engl J Med* 2004;350:1953–9.
10. Chatterjee K, Massie B. Systolic and diastolic heart failure: differences and similarities. *J Card Fail* 2007;13:569–76.
11. Francis GS, Benedict C, Jonstone D, et al. Comparison of neuroendocrine activation in patients with left ventricular dysfunction with and without congestive heart failure. *Circulation* 1990;82:1724–9.
12. Rihal CS, Davis KB, Kennedy JW, et al. The utility of clinical, electrocardiographic, and roentgenographic variables in the prediction of left ventricular function. *Am J Cardiol* 1995;75:220–3.
13. McCullough PA, Nowak RM, McCord J, et al. B-type natriuretic peptide and clinical judgment in the emergency diagnosis of heart failure: analysis from the Breathing Not Properly (BNP) Multinational Study. *Circulation* 2002;106:416–22.
14. Maisel AS, Krishnaswamy P, Nowak RM, et al. Rapid measurement of B-type natriuretic peptide in the emergency diagnosis of heart failure. *N Engl J Med* 2002;347:161–7.
15. Botvinick EH, Glazer H, Shosa D. What is the reliablity and utility of scintigraphic methods for the assessment of ventricular function? *Cardiovasc Clin* 1983;13:65–90.
16. Bonow RR, Bacharach SL, Green MV, et al. Impaired left ventricular diastolic filling in patients with coronary artery disease: assessment with radionuclide angiography. *Circulation* 1981;64:315–23.
17. Nieminen MS, Bohm M, Cowie MR, et al. Executive summary of the guidelines on the diagnosis and treatment of acute heart failure: the Task Force on Acute Heart Failure of the European Society of Cardiology. *Eur Heart J* 2005;26:384–416.
18. Cleland JG, Swedberg K, Follath F, et al. The EuroHeart Failure survey programme – a survey on the quality of care among patients with heart failure in Europe. Part 1: patient characteristics and diagnosis. *Eur Heart J* 2003;24:442–63.
19. Cowie MR, Wood DA, Coats AJ, et al. Incidence and aetiology of heart failure; a population-based study. *Eur Heart J* 1999;20:421–8.
20. Yancy CW, Lopatin M, Stevenson LW, et al. Clinical presentation, management, and in-hospital outcomes of patients admitted with acute decompensated heart failure with preserved systolic function: a report from the Acute Decompensated Heart Failure National Registry (ADHERE) Database. *J Am Coll Cardiol* 2006;47:76–84.
21. Fox KA, Steg PG, Eagle KA, et al. Decline in rates of death and heart failure in acute coronary syndromes, 1999–2006. *JAMA* 2007;297:1892–1900.
22. Cowie MR, Fox KF, Wood DA, et al. Hospitalization of patients with heart failure: a population-based study. *Eur Heart J* 2002;23:877–85.
23. Thom T, Haase N, Rosamond W, et al. Heart disease and stroke statistics – 2006 update: a report from the American Heart Association Statistics Committee and Stroke Statistics Subcommittee. *Circulation* 2006;113:e85–151.
24. Cowie MR, Mosterd A, Wood DA, et al. The epidemiology of heart failure. *Eur Heart J* 1997;18:208–25.
25. Mendez GF, Cowie MR. The epidemiological features of heart failure in developing countries: a review of the literature. *Int J Cardiol* 2001;80:213–19.
26. Levy D, Kenchaiah S, Larson MG, et al. Long-term trends in the incidence of and survival with heart failure. *N Engl J Med* 2002;347:1397–402.

27. Senni M, Tribouilloy CM, Rodeheffer RJ, et al. Congestive heart failure in the community: trends in incidence and survival in a 10-year period. *Arch Intern Med* 1999;159:29–34.

28. Barker WH, Mullooly JP, Getchell W. Changing incidence and survival for heart failure in a well-defined older population, 1970–1974 and 1990–1994. *Circulation* 2006;113:799–805.

29. Kannel WB, Castelli WP, McNamara PM, et al. Role of blood pressure in the development of congestive heart failure. The Framingham Study. *N Engl J Med* 1972;287:781–7.

30. Ho KK, Pinsky JL, Kannel WB, et al. The epidemiology of heart failure: the Framingham Study. *J Am Coll Cardiol* 1993;22(4 Suppl. A):6A–13A.

31. Fox KF, Cowie MR, Wood DA, et al. Coronary artery disease as the cause of incident heart failure in the population. *Eur Heart J* 2001;22:228–36.

32. Eriksson H, Svardsudd K, Larsson B, et al. Risk factors for heart failure in the general population: the study of men born in 1913. *Eur Heart J* 1989;10:647–56.

33. Kenchaiah S, Evans JC, Levy D, et al. Obesity and the risk of heart failure. *N Engl J Med* 2002;347:305–13.

34. Berry C, Murdoch DR, McMurray JJ. Economics of chronic heart failure. *Eur J Heart Fail* 2001;3:283–91.

35. McMurray JJ, Petrie MC, Murdoch DR, et al. Clinical epidemiology of heart failure: public and private health burden. *Eur Heart J* 1998;19(Suppl. P):P9–16.

36. McAlister FA, Stewart S, Ferrua S, et al. Multidisciplinary strategies for the management of heart failure patients at high risk for admission: a systematic review of randomized trials. *J Am Coll Cardiol* 2004;44:810–19.

37. The Scandinavian Simvastatin Survival Study Group. Randomised trial of cholesterol lowering in 4444 patients with coronary heart disease: the Scandinavian Simvastatin Survival Study (4S). *Lancet* 1994;344:1383–9.

38. Folkeringa RJ, Van Kraaij DV, Tieleman RG, et al. Statins associated with reduced mortality in patients admitted for congestive heart failure. *J Card Fail* 2006;12:134–8.

39. Cohn JN, Archibald DG, Ziesche S, et al. Effect of vasodilator therapy on mortality in chronic congestive heart failure. Results of a Veterans Administration Cooperative Study. *N Engl J Med* 1986;314:1547–52.

40. Cohn JN, Johnson G, Ziesche S, et al. A comparison of enalapril with hydralazine-isosorbide dinitrate in the treatment of chronic congestive heart failure *N Engl J Med* 1991;325:303–10.

41. Taylor AL, Ziesche S, Yancy C, et al. Combination of isosorbide dinitrate and hydralazine in blacks with heart failure. *N Engl J Med* 2004;351:2049–57.

42. Garg R, Yusuf S. Overview of randomized trials of angiotensin-converting enzyme inhibitors on mortality and morbidity in patients with heart failure. Collaborative Group on ACE Inhibitor Trials. *JAMA* 1995;273:1450–6.

43. The CONSENSUS Trial Study Group. Effects of enalapril on mortality in severe congestive heart failure. Results of the Cooperative North Scandinavian Enalapril Survival Study (CONSENSUS). *N Engl J Med* 1987;316:1429–35.

44. The SOLVD investigators. Effect of enalapril on survival in patients with reduced left ventricular ejection fractions and congestive heart failure. *N Engl J Med* 1991;325:293–302.

45. Pfeffer MA, Braunwald E, Moy LA, et al. Effect of captopril on mortality and morbidity in patients with left-ventricular dysfunction after myocardial infarction: results of the survival and ventricular enlargement trial. *N Engl J Med* 1992;327:669–77.

46. Shibata MC, Flather MD, Wang D. Systematic review of the impact of beta blockers on mortality and hospital admissions in heart failure. *Eur J Heart Fail* 2001;3:351–7.

47. Packer M, Coats AJ, Fowler MB, et al Carvedilol Prospective Randomized Cumulative Survival Study Group. Effect of carvedilol on survival in severe chronic heart failure. *N Engl J Med* 2001;344:1651–8.

48. Hjalmarson A, Goldstein S, Fagerberg B, et al. Effects of controlled-release metoprolol on total mortality, hospitalizations and well-being in patients with heart failure: the Metoprolol CR/XL Randomized Intervention Trial in congestive heart failure (MERIT-HF). *JAMA* 2000;283:1295–302.

49. CIBIS-II Investigators and Committees. The Cardiac Insufficiency Bisoprolol Study (CIBIS-II): a randomized trial. *Lancet* 1999;353:9–13.

50. Poole-Wilson PA, Swedberg K, Cleland JG, et al. Comparison of carvedilol and metoprolol on clinical outcomes in patients with chronic heart failure in the Carvedilol Or Metoprolol European Trial (COMET): randomized controlled trial. *Lancet* 2003;362:7–13.

51. Pitt B, Poole-Wilson PA, Segal R, et al. Effect of losartan compared with captopril on mortality in patients with symptomatic heart failure: randomised trial – the Losartan Heart Failure Survival Study ELITE II. *Lancet* 2000;355:1582–7.

52. Cohn JN, Tognoni G. Valsartan Heart Failure Trial Investigators. A randomized trial of the angiotensin-receptor blocker valsartan in chronic heart failure. *N Engl J Med* 2001;345:1667–75.

53. Granger CB, McMurray JJ, Yusuf S, et al. for the CHARM Investigators and Committees. Effects of candesartan in patients with chronic heart failure and reduced left-ventricular systolic function intolerant to angiotensin-converting-enzyme inhibitors: the CHARM-alternative trial. *Lancet* 2003;362:772–6.

54. McMurray JJ, Ostergren J, Swedberg K, et al. Effects of candesartan in patients with chronic heart failure and reduced left-ventricular systolic function taking angiotensin-converting-enzyme inhibitors: the CHARM-Added trial. *Lancet* 2003;362:767–71.

55. The Digitalis Investigation Group. The effect of digoxin on mortality and morbidity in patients with heart failure. *N Engl J Med* 1997;336:525–33.

56. O'Connor CM, Gattis WA, Uretsky BF, et al. Continuous intravenous dobutamine is associated with an increased risk of death in patients with advanced heart failure: insights from the Flolan International Randomized Survival Trial (FIRST). *Am Heart J* 1999;138:78–86.

57. Pitt B, Zannad F, Remme WJ, et al. The effect of spironolactone on mortality and morbidity in patients with severe heart failure. *N Engl J Med* 1999;341:709–17.

58. Thackray S, Witte K, Clark AL, et al. Clinical trials update: OPTIME-CHF, PRAISE-2, ALL-HAT. *Eur J Heart Fail* 2000;2:209–12.

59. Remme WJ, Swedberg K for the Task Force for the Diagnosis and Treatment of Chronic Heart Failure, European Society of Cardiology. Guidelines for the diagnosis and treatment of chronic heart failure. *Eur Heart J* 2001;22:1527–60.

60. Allman KC, Shaw LJ, Hachamovitch R, et al. Myocardial viability testing and impact of revascularization on prognosis in patients with coronary artery disease and left ventricular dysfunction: a meta-analysis. *J Am Coll Cardiol* 2002;39:1151–8.

61. Cleland JG, Daubert JC, Erdmann E, et al. for the Cardiac Resynchronization-Heart Failure (CARE-HF) Study Investigators. The effect of cardiac resynchronization on morbidity and mortality in heart failure. *N Engl J Med* 2005;352:1539–49.

62. Bristow MR, Saxon LA, Boehmer J, et al. Cardiac resynchronization therapy with or without an implantable defibrillator in advanced chronic heart failure. *N Engl J Med* 2004;350:2140–50.

63. Bardy GH, Lee KL, Mark DB, et al. Amiodarone or an implantable cardioverter-defibrillator for congestive heart failure. *N Engl J Med* 2005;352:225–37.

64. Moss A, Zareba W, Hall WJ, et al. Prophylactic implantation of a defibrillator in patients with myocardial infarction and reduced ejection fraction. *N Engl J Med* 2002;346:877–83.

65. Rose EA, Gelijns AC, Moskowitz AJ, et al. for the Randomized Evaluation of Mechanical Assistance for the Treatment of Congestive Heart Failure (REMATCH) Study Group. Long-term mechanical left ventricular assistance for end-stage heart failure. *N Engl J Med* 2001;345:1435–43.

66. Feldman AM, Silver MA, Francis GS, et al. for the PEECH Investigators. Enhanced external counterpulsation improves exercise tolerance in patients with chronic heart failure. *J Am Coll Cardiol* 2006;48:1198–205.

67. Taylor DO, Edwards LB, Boucek MM, et al. Registry of the International Society for Heart and Lung Transplantation: twenty-fourth official adult heart transplantation report – 2007. *J Heart Lung Transplant* 2007;26;769–81.

68. Yusuf S, Pfeffer MA, Swedberg K, et al. Effects of candesartan in patients with chronic heart failure and preserved ejection fraction: the CHARM-Preserved Trial. *Lancet* 2003;362:777–81.

69. Redfield MM, Jacobson SJ, Burnett JC Jr, et al. Burden of systolic and diastolic ventricular dysfunction in the community: appreciating the scope of the heart failure epidemic. *JAMA* 2003;289:194–202.

70. McDonagh TA, Morrison CE, Lawrence A, et al. Symptomatic and asymptomatic left-ventricular systolic dysfunction in an urban population. *Lancet* 1997;350:829–33.

71. Cowie MR, Wood DA, Coats AJ, et al. Survival of patients with a new diagnosis of heart failure: a population based study. *Heart* 2000;83:505–10.

72. Quinn M, Babb P, Brock A, et al. *Cancer trends in England and Wales, 1950–1999: Studies on Medical and Population Subjects No.66.* London: Office for National Statistics, 2001.

73. Roughton M, Mannam I, Sutton GC, et al. Long term survival of patients with a new diagnosis of heart failure: a population based prospective cohort study. *Heart* 2007;93(Suppl. 1):85 (abstr.).

74. Roger VL, Weston SA, Redfield MM, et al. Trends in heart failure incidence and survival in a community-based population. *JAMA* 2004;292:344–50.

75. Mehta PA, Dubrey SW, McIntyre HF, et al. Improved survival for patients with incident heart failure in the UK population. *Eur Heart J* 2006;27:51 (abstr.).

76. Mosterd A, Cost B, Hoes AW, et al. The prognosis of heart failure in the general population: The Rotterdam Study. *Eur Heart J* 2001;22:1318–27.

77. Solomon S, Olofsson B, Finn P, et al. Cause of death across full spectrum of ventricular function in patients with heart failure: the CHARM study. *J Am Coll Cardiol* 2004;43(Suppl. 1):180 (abstr.).

78. Owan TE, Hodge DO, Herges RM, et al. Trends in prevalence and outcome of heart failure with preserved ejection fraction. *N Engl J Med* 2006;355:251–9.

Abbreviations

ACE	angiotensin-converting enzyme
ARB	angiotensin II receptor blocker
BNP	B-type natriuretic peptide
CAD	coronary artery disease
CRT	cardiac resynchronization therapy
CT	computed tomography
DC	direct current
ECG	electrocardiogram
EECP	enhanced external counterpulsation
EF	ejection fraction
IABP	intra-aortic balloon counterpulsation
ICD	implantable cardioverter-defibrillator
IV	intravenous
LV	left ventricular
MI	myocardial infarction
MMP	matrix metalloproteinase
MRI	magnetic resonance imaging
NSTEMI	non-ST-segment elevation myocardial infarction
PCI	percutaneous coronary intervention
STEMI	ST-segment elevation myocardial infarction
TIMP	tissue inhibitor of metalloproteinase

Index

Page numbers in **bold** refer to figures; those in *italics* refer to tables.

A

ACE inhibitors *see* angiotensin-converting enzyme inhibitors
activation, neurohormonal 8–9, **8**, **9**
acute coronary syndromes, management of
    ACE inhibitors and ARBs 36
    with β-blockers 36
    high mortality of patients 36
    percutaneous coronary intervention 36
    surgical intervention 36–7
Acute Decompensated Heart Failure National Registry
    (ADHERE) 32
acute heart failure
    bilateral crackles of lungs 11
    cardiac abnormality responsible for **2**, 11, **11**
    epidemiologic information 30
    impaired perfusion of vital organs 11
    investigations *see* acute heart failure investigations
    management of *see* acute heart failure,
        management of
    mitral valves 11, **11**
    pulsus alternans 11, **11**
    symptoms of 10
acute heart failure investigations
    B-type natriuretic peptide 16, **16**
    plain chest X-ray 15, **15**
    resting electrocardiogram 15, **15**, **16**
acute heart failure, management of *37*
    acute coronary syndromes 36–7
    arrhythmias 35–6
    eliminating pulmonary edema 34–5 *see also*
        pulmonary edema, treatment of
    improving organ perfusion 35
    maintaining adequate oxygenation 34
acute myocardial infarction 5, 6, 8, *15*, 30
ADHERE *see* Acute Decompensated Heart Failure
    National Registry
advanced heart failure
    atrial fibrillation *13*, 17
    cardiac output 28
    myocyte loss in 7
    nonpharmacologic treatment of 47
    pulmonary hypertension 28
    vasodilators 38, **38**
advanced heart failure, management of 47
    cardiac transplantation 47, *47*
    conventional surgical treatment 43
    device treatments 43–6
aldosterone inhibitors 37, 42, **42**, *43*

amiloride 38
amiodarone
    antiarrhythmic agent 42
    for atrial flutter 35
    for chronic heart failure with reduced EF 47
    decreasing frequency of ICD discharge 43, 45
    preventing recurrence 36
    sinus rhythm, maintaining of 35
    slowing rapid heart rate 47
    versus ICD therapy 45, **46**
angiotensin-converting enzyme (ACE) inhibitors
    asymptomatic LV systolic dysfunction 39, **39**
    for chronic heart failure *43*
    comparative trial with ARBs 40–1
    improving prognosis and mortality rates 38, 39,
        39, 48
    incompatibility with aspirin therapy 43
    patients with acute MI and 36
    pharmacologic agents 37, 43
    restriction by unwanted effects 40
angiotensin II receptor blockers (ARBs)
    combination therapy with ACE inhibitors 40–1
    patients with acute MI and 36
    pharmacologic agent 37
    reducing mortality and morbidity 40–1, **41**, 47
antiarrhythmic agents
    amiodarone 42
    catheter-based ablation therapy 42
    Class III drugs 42
    pharmacologic treatment of chronic heart failure
        43, *43*
anticoagulants
    arrhythmias, management and 36
    as pharmacologic agent 37
    for chronic heart failure 43, *43*
ARBs *see* angiotensin II receptor blockers
arrhythmia, management of 35
    anticoagulation 36
    direct current cardioversion 36
    pacemaker, insertion of 36
atrial fibrillation
    in advanced heart failure 17
    amiodarone curing 47, *47*
    anticoagulation curing 36, 43
    catheter-based ablation therapy 42
    common finding in chronic heart failure 13, **13**, 42
    development of acute heart failure 11, 15, 30, 35
    digitalis preparations curing 41
    direct current cardioversion 35
    exacerbation of heart failure and 10, 14, **14**, 15

    palpitation and 12
    raising B-type natriuretic peptide levels *20*

B

B-type natriuretic peptide (BNP)
    for acute heart failure 16, **16**
    for chronic heart failure 19–20, **20**
    raising levels of, conditions for *20*
bisoprolol 40, **40**
β-blockers
    for MI patients 36
    for controlling ventricular rate in atrial fibrillation
        47, *47*
    for management of arrhythmias 35
    as pharmacologic agent 37
    in pharmacologic treatment of chronic heart
        failure *43*
    for reducing mortality 40, **40**, 48
    for reducing sudden cardiac death 40
BNP *see* B-type natriuretic peptide
breathlessness
    ACE inhibitors curing 39
    in acute heart failure 10
    cardiac or noncardiac cause for 19, 20
    caused by pulmonary congestion 10
    in chronic heart failure 11
    in exacerbated heart failure 14
    loop diuretics 34, 38
    morphine or diamorphine curing 34
    normal BNP level 16, **16**
    symptom of heart failure 1
bumetanide and diuretic treatment 38

C

CAD *see* coronary artery disease
calcium-channel blockers 37, 42, *43*, 47
candesartan 41, **41**
captopril **39**
cardiac abnormalities
    evidence of 2, **2**
    investigations for 3 *see also* invasive and
        noninvasive investigations
cardiac resynchronization therapy (CRT)
    combined treatment with ICD and 44, **45**
    nuclear techniques for diagnosis and 26, **26**

patients with chronic heart failure and preserved EF, role in 47

patients with heart failure with reduced EF 43–4, **44**

patients with mechanical dyssynchrony 44, 45

cardiac transplantation 47, **47**

carvedilol 40, **40**

catheterization 27–8, **27**, **28**, **29** *see also* investigations into etiology of heart failure

chronic heart failure

abnormal physical signs in patient 2, 12–13, **12**

atrial fibrillation 13, **13**

breathlessness, mechanism of 11–12

epidemiologic information on 31 *see also* epidemiologic information

fatigue 12

management of *see* chronic heart failure, management of

investigations *see* chronic heart failure investigations

with preserved ejection fraction, management of 47, *47*

symptoms of 11, 12

chronic heart failure investigations

exercise testing 20, **20**

natriuretic peptides 19–20, **20**, *20*

plain chest X-ray 16, **17**

resting electrocardiogram 17, **18**, **19**

chronic heart failure, management of

pharmacologic treatment *see* pharmacologic treatment for chronic heart failure

risk factor management 37

specialized support services 37

chronic heart failure with preserved EF, management of 47, *47*

computed tomography (CT) 26 *see also* investigations into etiology of heart failure

CONSENSUS *see* Cooperative North Scandinavian Enalapril Survival Study

conventional surgical treatments for advanced heart failure

aneurysmectomy 43

revascularization 43

Cooperative North Scandinavian Enalapril Survival Study (CONSENSUS) 39

coronary arteriography 29, **29** *see also* investigations into etiology of heart failure

coronary artery disease (CAD)

aspirin therapy 43

cause of heart disease 32

coronary arteriography in patients with **29**

myocardial dysfunction and 3

patients with 20, **25**, **28**

result of 5, 12, 14, 17, 25–6

risks factors for patients with 37

CRT *see* cardiac resynchronization therapy

CT *see* computed tomography

D

device treatments for advanced heart failure

cardiac resynchronization therapy 43–5, **44**, **45**

enhanced external counterpulsation 46

implantable cardioverter-defibrillator 45, **46**

LV assist devices 46

digitalis preparations

improving organ perfusion 35

positive inotropic action 35, 41, 43

treating atrial fibrillation 35, *47*

digoxin 41, 47

dipyridamole sestamibi 43

diuretics

ACE inhibitors and 40

breathlessness and fatigue 38

eliminating pulmonary edema 34–5, *37*

exacerbation of heart failure with change of *15*

fluid retention and 38, 47, *47*

pharmacologic treatment of chronic heart failure 37, 38, *43*

dobutamine

positive inotropic agent 35, 41

stress echocardiography 43

dofetilide 42

dopamine

positive ionotropic agent 41

vasopressor agent 35

dyspnea *see* breathlessness

E

eccentric hypertrophy 5

ECG *see* electrocardiogram

echocardiography and Doppler

apical wall motion abnormality **21**

decreased E to A wave ratio 22, **22**

enlargement of left atrium **21**

establishing cause of heart failure 21–22

E to A wave ratio consistent with restrictive physiology 22, **23**

hypertrophied left ventricle 22, **23**

idiopathic dilated cardiomyopathy **21**

mitral regurgitation 22, **22**

right ventricular hypertrophy and dilatation 23, **24**

transmitral flow patterns 22

tricuspid regurgitation 23, **24**

EECP *see* enhanced external counterpulsation (EECP)

EF *see* ejection fraction (EF)

ejection fraction (EF) 3

remodeling with preserved *see* pathophysiology of remodeling with preserved EF

remodeling with reduced *see* pathophysiology of remodeling with reduced EF

electrocardiogram (ECG)

in acute heart failure 15, **15**, **16**

in chronic heart failure 17, **18**, **19**

enhanced external counterpulsation (EECP) 43, 46, **47**

enoximone 35, 41

epidemiologic information

on acute heat failure 30

on age and sex 31, **32**

on chronic heart failure 31

cost of heart failure 33, **33**

on etiology of heart 32

on exacerbated heart failure 30–1

obesity 33

on prevalence and incidence of heart failure 31

epidemiologic information on acute heart failure 30

epidemiologic information on chronic heart failure 31

epidemiologic information on exacerbated heart failure 30–1

etiology of heart failure *see* investigations into etiology of heart failure

European Society of Cardiology

definition of heart failure 1

guidelines 30

exacerbated heart failure

definition of 14

epidemiological information on 30–1

factors causing 14, **14**, *15*

investigations 20 *see* acute heart failure investigations; chronic heart failure investigations

exercise testing 20, **20**

F

fluid retention

in patients with chronic heart failure 12

in patients with compensated heart failure 14

pharmacologic treatment 37 *see also* pharmacologic treatment for chronic heart failure

signs of heart failure 1

frusemide *see* furosemide

furosemide 38

G

gadolinium 26

H

heart failure

acute *see* acute heart failure

advanced *see* advanced heart failure

age and sex 31, **32**

cardiac abnormalities 2–3, **2**

chronic *see* chronic heart failure

classification of 10

cost of 33, **33**

definitions of 1

epidemiology 30–3

etiology of 32 *see also* investigations into etiology of heart failure

exacerbation of *see* exacerbated heart failure

functional abnormality in patients with overt 7

investigations of 15 *see also* invasive and noninvasive investigation

managing *see* heart failure management

myocardial dysfunction with preserved EF causing 6–7

myocardial dysfunction with reduced EF causing 4– 5

neurohormonal activation 8–9, **8**, **9**

obesity and 33

and pathophysiology *see* pathophysiology of heart failure

prevalence and incidence of 31

prognosis of *see* prognosis of heart failure

symptoms and signs 1

heart failure investigations

acute *see* acute heart failure investigations

chronic *see* chronic heart failure investigations

etiology of heat failure *see* investigations into etiology of heart failure

exacerbated *see* acute heart failure investigations; chronic heart failure investigations

heart failure management
managing acute heart failure 34–7 *see also* acute heart failure, management of
managing advanced heart failure 43–7 *see also* advanced heart failure, management of
managing chronic heart failure 37–43 *see also* chronic heart failure, management of
managing chronic heart failure with preserved EF 47, *47*
hemodynamic abnormalities
cardiac catheterization 27, **27**
cardiac output 28
coronary arteriography 29, **29**
reduced or preserved EF 28, **28**
variability of 28
hydralazine 38, **38**
hypertension
CAD and 32, 37
in chronic heart failure with preserved EF 47, *47*
common cause of heart failure 31, 32
exacerbation of heart failure and 15, *15*
pulmonary 23, *24*, 28, **28**
systemic 22, **23**

I

IABP *see* intra-aortic balloon counterpulsation
ICD *see* implantable cardioverter-defibrillator
implantable cardioverter-defibrillator (ICD)
combined treatment with CRT and 44
comparative trial of amiodarone or placebo with 45, *46*
nonpharmcologic treatment for advanced heart failure 43, *47*
in paroxysmal ventricular tachycardia 43
in ventricular arrhythmias 36
inotropic agents 35, 37, *37*, 41, 43
intra-aortic balloon counterpulsation (IABP) 36
invasive and noninvasive investigations
for acute heart failure *see* acute heart failure investigations
cardiac catheterization and coronary arteriography 27–9, **27**, **28**, **29**
for chronic heart failure *see* chronic heart failure investigations
echocardiography and Doppler 20–4 *see also* echocardiography and Doppler
MRI and CT, use of 26–27, **26**
myocardial biopsy 29, **29**
nuclear techniques 25–6 *see also* nuclear techniques
investigations into etiology of heart failure
cardiac catheterization 27, **27**
CT, use of 26
coronary arteriography 29, **29**
dilated cardiomyopathy 28, **29**
echocardiography and Doppler *see also* echocardiography and Doppler
hemodynamic changes in patients 28
impaired systolic function 28
localized hypokinesis/LV dilatation 28, **28**
LV angiography 28
magnetic resonance imaging 26, **27**
myocardial biopsy 29, **29**
nuclear techniques 25–6, **25**, **26**
isosorbide dinitrate 38, **38**

L

left ventricular assist devices 43, 46, *47*
left ventricular myocardial disease 3, 10
left ventricular remodeling 4
neurohormonal activation 8–9, **8**, **9**
with preserved ejection fraction 6–8 *see also* pathophysiology of remodeling with preserved EF
with reduced ejection fraction 4–6, **4**, *4 see also* pathophysiology of remodeling with reduced EF
left ventricular systolic function 8–9, **8**, **9**
levosimendan 35
Lewis, Thomas 1
loop diuretics 34, 35, 38

M

magnetic resonance imaging (MRI) 26, **27**
matrix metalloproteinase (MMP) 5
metoprolol 40
MI *see* myocardial infarction (MI)
milrinone 35, 41
MMP *see* matrix metalloproteinase
MRI *see* magnetic resonance imaging
myocardial biopsy 29, **29** *see also* investigations into etiology of heart failure
myocardial disease
classification of 10
LV 3
with preserved EF 6, 7
with reduced EF 5, 20
myocardial dysfunction 3, 4–7
myocardial infarction (MI) **3**, **4**, **15**, **18** *see also* acute myocardial infarction
myocardium 4, 26, 29, 43, *47*

N

natriuretic peptides
in acute heart failure 16, **16**
in chronic heart failure 19–20, **20**, *20*
neurohormonal activation
following acute myocardial infarction 8, **8**
in heart failure with reduced and preserved EF 8, 9, **9**
mechanisms responsible for 8
producing adverse ventricular and vascular remodeling 9
vicious cycles of heart failure 8–9, **9**
nitroglycerine 35, 38
non-ST-segment MI (NSTEMI) 36
norepinephrine 9, 35
NSTEMI *see* non-ST-segment MI
nuclear techniques
chronic ischemia of the myocardium 26, **26**
equilibrium phase 25, **25**
parameters of diastolic function 25, **25**
positron emission tomography 26, **26**
radionuclide ventriculography 25, 26, **26**
technetium-90m labeling 25
thallium-201 imaging 26, 43

O

organ perfusion improvement 35
oxygenation, maintenance of adequate 34

P

pathophysiology of heart failure
chronic constrictive pericarditis **4**
comparison of principal differences of reduced EF and preserved EF 7, *7*
development of secondary mitral regurgitation 4
localized LV aneurysm **3**
LV remodeling *see* left ventricular remodeling
major functional abnormality in patients 7, *7*, **8**
neurohormonal activation 8–9, **8**, **9**
partial avulsion of papillary muscle **4**
pathological conditions of heart 3–4, *3*, **4**
remodeling with preserved EF *see* pathophysiology of remodeling with preserved EF
remodeling with reduced EF *see* pathophysiology of remodeling with reduced EF
right ventricular view in tetralogy of Fallot **4**
transverse slice of ventricles **3**
pathophysiology of remodeling with preserved EF 6, *6*, **6**
causing exacerbations of heart failure 14, *14*
diastolic pressure–volume curve 7, **8**
disproportionate increase in LV diastolic pressure 7, *7*
functional abnormality in patients 7
heart failure with 5
neurohormonal activation 8–9, **8**
normal EF of LV wall thickness 6
systolic pressure–volume curve **8**
thicker collagen fibrillar bundles **5**, *7*
tissue expressions of MMPs and TIMPs 7
pathophysiology of remodeling with reduced EF *4*
eccentric hypertrophy 5, **5**
LV biopsy 5
mechanical dyssynchrony 4
mechanisms of 5
neurohormonal values in patients 8–9, **9**
shape change of left ventricle 4, **4**
specific remodeling features 5, **6**
PCI *see* percutaneous coronary intervention
percutaneous coronary intervention (PCI) 36
pharmacologic treatment for chronic heart failure 37, *43*
ACE inhibitors 39–40, **39**
aldosterone inhibitors 42, **42**
antiarrhythmic agents 42–3
anticoagulants 43
ARBs 40–1, **41**
β-blockers 40, *40*
calcium-channel blockers 42
digitalis preparations 41
diuretics 38
positive inotropic agents 41–2
vasodilators 38, **38**
phenylephrine 35
plain chest X-ray
in acute heart failure 15, *15*
in chronic heart failure 16, *17*
positive inotropic agents
digitalis 41

other 41–2
prognosis of heart failure
    adverse prognostic features *48*
    individuals with systolic dysfunction with reduced
        EF *48*
    modes of death in patients with chronic heart failure
        49, **49**
    patients with heart failure, LV dysfunction, reduced
        EF 48, **49**
    patients with heart failure, LV dysfunction, preserved
        EF *50*
pulmonary edema, treatment of
    intravenous use of loop diuretics and 34–5
    morphine or diamorphine 34
    nitroglycerine and nitrates 35

R

resting electrocardiogram
    in acute heart failure 15, **15**, **16**
    in chronic heart failure 17–19, **18**, **19**

S

sodium nitroprusside
    eliminating pulmonary edema 35, *37*
    surgical intervention and 36
SOLVD trial *see* Studies of Left Ventricular Dysfunction trial
sotalol 42
spironolactone 42, **42**
ST-segment elevation MI (STEMI) 36
STEMI *see* ST-segment elevation MI
Studies of Left Ventricular Dysfunction trial 39

T

thallium-201 imaging 26, 43
technetium-90m labeling 25
thiazide diuretics 35, 38
TIMP *see* tissue inhibitor of metalloproteinase (TIMP)
tissue inhibitor of metalloproteinase (TIMP) 5
torasemide 38
torsemide *see* torasemide

V

vasodilators
    calcium-channel blockers as 42
    for improving mortality rates 38, **38**, 42
    for improving quality of life 38, **38**
    pharmacologic treatment by using 37, *43*
    for reducing acute pulmonary congestion 38